"Rolfer Noah Karrasch—recognizing that the line between therapist and client is a thin one indeed—has written a book that would serve either consumer or provider in reaching below the surface to the psychological and expressive correlates that nearly always accompany postural pain/strain patterns. So many somatic psychology books are psychobabble with a smattering of the body th̶ ̶ ̶ ̶ ̶ ̶'̶ ̶m.' By contrast, this book starts with t̶ ̶ ̶ ̶ ̶givi̶ ̶ ̶ ̶ ̶v in to authentic self-ex

*Maine, USA*

"Combining ̶ ̶ ̶ ̶ ̶ ̶ ̶ ̶ ̶ ̶ ̶ ̶ ̶ ̶ ̶ ̶ ̶ ̶ ̶ ̶ ̶ ̶ ̶ ̶ ̶ ̶ork, Noah brings a blend of ancient and modern thought to his bodywork approach. Littered with useful and provocative images and exercises, this book will help a therapist get to many of their clients' 'core' issues by contacting both the emotional and the physical aspects of pain. A worthy addition to any bodyworker's bookshelf."

—*James Earls BA (Hons Psych), Structural Integration Practitioner, author of* Fascial Release for Structural Balance, *and Director of Kinesis UK*

"Just as a skilled bodywork session should speak to all the layers and unite the disparate energies of the body, *Freeing Emotions and Energy Through Myofascial Release* brilliantly unites the specific manual techniques and structural theory of a holistic bodywork session with the deeper psychological and emotional understanding of not only our clients, but of our own processes. In this fine book, Noah Karrasch moves knowledge to the next plateau of wisdom."

—*Art Riggs, Advanced Certified Rolfer, international teacher, and author of* Deep Tissue Massage

"*Freeing Emotions and Energy Through Myofascial Release* expands our awareness of the many ways we get 'stuck' in the flow of our lives. I'm fascinated by the powerful parallel of this work with Interactive Imagery and Biofeedback, and encouraged at the multiple avenues we have to be HEALTHY ̶ ̶ ̶ ̶ ̶ ̶NS While respecting our emotions, we can release 'stuck' and move

—*Patricia Pike, Guided Imagery and Biofeedback Practitioner, ̶*

"*Freeing Emotions and Energy Through Myofascial Release* is an imme book for everyone who wants to be alive, fully alive. It is a p to health and emotional freedom, integrating models from F into an empowering vision of how free and unblocked we can dare to."

—*Michael Kaufmann, NLP Practitio* *and meditation tea*

"For many people, especially physicians and health care providers, discussions about chakras and Chinese healing concepts are so far out of our frame of reference, and so far out of our knowledge and experience, that it is something that we avoid. In this book, Noah brings together in a 'physical way' relating or connecting the chakras and traditional Chinese medicine with physical human anatomy. Now, I can picture the concepts, and begin a process of integrating traditional Western and Eastern forms of healing. He also 'brings a challenge' to each healer, regardless of our title, to go deeper into the core structure and function of the person—combining the dimensions of physical, emotional, intellectual, and spiritual self. It is a 'good read,' but also an enlightening and refreshing view of the integrated whole person."

—*Ralph Harvey, MD, Cornerstone Family Practice, PLC, Associate Professor, Michigan State University College of Human Medicine, USA*

"I first came to know of Noah through a mutual friend who recommended I meet this 'American therapist' who had a different approach to soft tissue work. Over the years he has shared those views with many of my students who have all come away from his classes both enriched and inspired. I have witnessed his generosity of spirit, his compassion for those he serves, and it is reflected in this gem of a book. He has brought together a philosophy that in essence has been around for a long time, but not connected in a way in which Noah has been able to demonstrate. Follow his journey, make it yours, it will bring a new dimension to your treatments as well as yourself. I have witnessed his generosity of spirit, his compassion for those he serves, and it is reflected in this gem of a book. He has brought together a philosophy that in essence has been around for a long time, but not connected in a way in which Noah has been able to demonstrate. Follow his journey, make it yours, it will bring a new dimension to your treatments as well as yourself."

—*Susan Findlay, BSc RGN, Dip SMRT, MSMA MLCSP, MCNHC, Director of North London School of Sports Massage, UK*

"Hugely informative, easily accessible to bodyworker, student and receiver alike. Everyone will come away with something useful."

—*Bev Breeze, Shiatsu Practitioner and instructor, London, UK*

"My coffee sat cold on the counter as I paged through. It's exciting to see a book written about putting the spirit back in bodywork both for the client and the therapist. YES. I love the way you have blended your CORE Fascial Release Bodywork with the chakra system as you think about the areas being worked on. Attention and Intention of both client and therapist working together. Perfect."

—*Brenda Messling, Massage Therapy instructor and teacher of Creative Healing, Arkansas, USA*

"As a Chartered Physiotherapist and Pilates teacher, Noah's CORE Fascial Release technique and its representation in this book have quite simply changed the way I work. It has helped to make complex cases simple, creating new parallels with the manual work used in Physiotherapy and the exercises prescribed in Pilates. *Freeing Emotions and Energy Through Myofascial Release* will aid any movement therapist to 'bridge the gaps' in their ability to deliver consistently successful therapy."

—*Robert White, Chartered Physiotherapist and Pilates teacher, and Director of Body2Fit, Stockton-on-Tees, UK*

"*Freeing Emotions and Energy Through Myofascial Release* is a compendium of classical structural bodywork principles, concepts from Oriental medicine, and psychological common sense. Noah Karrasch challenges healers of all disciplines to explore their own body-mind connections and disconnections in order to become more fully present with their clients. We are blessed to be beneficiaries of his 25 years of dedication to holistic healing."

—*Mary Bond, author of* The New Rules of Posture: How to Sit, Stand, and Move in the Modern World

# FREEING EMOTIONS AND ENERGY THROUGH MYOFASCIAL RELEASE

Noah Karrasch

Foreword by C. Norman Shealy, MD, PhD

Illustrated by Julie Zaslow and Amy Rizzo

SINGING
DRAGON

LONDON AND PHILADELPHIA

First published in 2012
by Singing Dragon
an imprint of Jessica Kingsley Publishers
116 Pentonville Road
London N1 9JB, UK
and
400 Market Street, Suite 400
Philadelphia, PA 19106, USA

*www.singingdragon.com*

**Library of Congress Cataloging in Publication Data**
Karrasch, Noah.
Freeing emotions and energy through myofascial release / Noah Karrasch ; foreword by C. Norman
Healy ; illustrated by Julie Zaslow and Amy Rizza.
p. cm.
Includes bibliographical references and index.
ISBN 978-1-84819-085-6 (alk. paper)
1. Mind and body therapies. 2. Manipulation (Therapeutics) I. Title.
RC489.M53K37 2012
615.8'52--dc23
2011029657

**British Library Cataloguing in Publication Data**
A CIP catalogue record for this book is available from the British Library

ISBN 978 1 84819 085 6
eISBN 978 0 85701 065 0

Printed and bound in Great Britain

*This book came about because of my realization, both during work with clients and in my personal life, that each individual essence needs and deserves to be unwound. As others discharge their hurts for us to nurture, we not only learn to respect and appreciate them more but we validate them in a way that makes us, and them, whole. As we approach this unity, we realize the most important trait to develop in our personal and larger world as well is, simply, gratitude. Hopefully, learning to be grateful will also teach us to want to be more responsible, generous, and caring in the larger world. And if we as practitioners, therapists, and friends can make this shift to being true to ourselves, we can more truly assist those around us in their journeys.*

*So, the book is dedicated to all—clients, family, colleagues, students, and teachers—who have helped me on this path and shown me that indeed every journey is a rich and deep story. I am grateful. Thank you to all my mirrors.*

# DISCLAIMER

This book is not meant to take the place of medical care, but to enhance it. It's designed primarily for therapists of every stripe who are interested in exploring how emotions create physical health or illness, and how physical health or illness contributes to emotional health.

# CONTENTS

# FOREWORD

*BY C. NORMAN SHEALY, MD, PHD*

I was first exposed to Rolfing in May 1974 and had three sessions in a week while attending The May Lectures in London. About a year later, I experienced the first full ten sessions of Rolfing and over the next year I had about ten more. I then met Ida Rolf and she said: "You are not supposed to become addicted to it!"

Actually in my original session 4 it hurt so much that I started laughing, thinking: "I can't believe I am paying this guy $60 to do this!" The Rolfer began laughing and it took us four hours to finish the session. I also had a very painful session with one of the Rolf Institute instructors, but from the beginning it was obvious that the day *after* a session I always felt terrific. Of course we did not know about beta endorphins until the early 1980s; we now know that a significant physically painful experience releases beta endorphins, the natural narcotics.

Because of multiple spinal injuries and surgeries, I have had many kinks in my body. In the early 1980s I had the great fortune to meet Noah Karrasch and began sessions with him. Overall, Noah's CORE sessions are far more gentle than those of other Rolfers I have experienced (counting my earlier experiences, a total of 78 sessions). Indeed, because of the tremendous benefit in function, I could become addicted! In the mid 1980s I happened to receive a phone call from Noah, who had just been involved in a plane crash in the South. He had suffered a spinal fracture and was partially paralyzed. I was able to assist him in returning to Springfield, Missouri, where he had appropriate surgery and a remarkable recovery. It was one of the great privileges of my life to assist Noah, who contributed so much to my own comfort.

Of course, Noah's experience also gave me much to ponder. I have always had a problem with the metaphysical concept that we attract our illnesses and accidents. Noah told me that he and the pilot friend had just spent two days griping about the fact that they gave and gave nurturing but never received. Their plane crashed because of a faulty fuel gauge which misled them into thinking it was one-quarter full when it was empty! Now he had to accept nurturing, which he did with gratitude and, of course, recovery. Synchronicity in action?

Personally, I believe the essential reason for life is to do good to others, to nurture them. Noah's CORE program is a tremendous evolution in the nurturing practice of fascial, muscle, tendon, and skeletal alignment. In this exciting new book, Noah goes well beyond the physical adjustments with practical exercises and the most important advice of all: Holding a grudge is like taking poison and expecting it to kill the other person. You cannot afford the luxury of anger, guilt, anxiety, or depression. Follow his CORE advice to optimal health.

*C. Norman Shealy, MD, PhD*
*President, Holos Institutes of Health*
*Founding President, American Holistic Medical Association*
*www.normshealy.com*

# ACKNOWLEDGMENTS

...to Ida Rolf, Louis Schultz, Stacey Mills, Emmett Hutchens, Byron Gentry, Wilhelm Reich, and John Pierrakos, only four of whom I had the pleasure to know.

...to my prayer partners of many years, Bee and Glo.

...to my colleagues past and present from whichever world who have shared ideas and work across the years.

...to my family for being the crucible in which these ideas have been transformed.

...to Jessica Kingsley for encouraging me to find my voice, and helping me make it stronger, clearer, and less insistent.

...to Bev Breeze who brought me the breath of fresh air her name would imply.

...to Patricia Pike, Bill Zaslow, and Gen Stacey whose reading of early manuscripts helped me realize what I wanted to say and how to say it more clearly.

...to Susan Findlay, Tom Myers, Ralph Harvey, Mary Bond, Art Riggs, and Martin Logue, who have provided valuable feedback for the final product.

...to students, friends, and clients who have taught me so much about myself and our work.

...to the Higher Power, Deepest Deep, One God who truly creates and cares for all, whether we accept this care or not. I believe God enjoys our praise and worship, but is truly thrilled with our gratitude.

And a special acknowledgment to the family:

...to John and Gertie, Pete and Lottie—my grandparents.

...to John and Elizabeth—my parents.

...to Anna Lou, Susan, Mary Lynn—my sisters.

...to Gloria and Jacki—my partners.

...to Molly and Andrew—my children.

...to Henry Atlas Wineberg and the as-yet-unborn and unnamed new generations—may their journeys be easier, but no less remarkable.

# TO THE THERAPIST

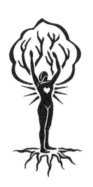

## TOUCHING THE CORE

*Whether dealing with physical, mental, or emotional pain
or blockage, it's important to reach inside and examine,
soften, and process to eliminate pains and fears.*

*If we can create space between groin, gut, heart,
and head, we're already healing.*

I'm going to challenge you to be a more effective and empathetic therapist, and I want you to take everything you read in this book with a grain of salt.

Years ago I read a quote along those lines that I'll paraphrase: "Beware of all proselytizing men, who tell you they have your answers...and beware of me also." I've always believed this made sense: What could be more foolish than allowing someone else to be your authority for *your* life, *your* decisions, and *your* body? It's simply wrong to look exclusively to external authorities, and I've striven to not become anyone's external authority.

And yet...what could be more foolish than *not* listening to and exposing yourself to different ideas, both common knowledge and common sense? We know when we're sick we need a doctor; but common sense often lets us take care of our own problems by slowing down and getting rest instead of finding an outside expert. Knowledge sometimes has lost—or hasn't yet discovered—its common sense.

Much of what you read in this book is my observation and common sense; some of it may seem at odds with common knowledge. If you require data and research to validate knowledge, you'll possibly be amused at or even scornful of some of my observations. My body has been my laboratory for a long time. If you'll accept that 25 years of pursuing the bodywork craft in an injured body *is* research, I believe you'll find new ideas to ponder and new ways to challenge clients to feel their bodies and free their emotions. Use your own discernment to decide which of my common sense, what I call *mywhy*, resonates for you, and what common knowledge you may want to rethink. My intention is to collect, blend, and share ageless common sense that allows you to experience your clients and their wounds in a new and hopefully useful way. I hope to help you see that you best facilitate healing in clients by helping them know themselves, and that to do so you must know yourself. A good practitioner looks and listens, then probes with words and touch.

I say "a good practitioner" because I believe the model is less important than the intention. I hope this book will serve not only deep tissue and massage therapists, but physical therapists, doctors, psychologists and counselors, Pilates and yoga instructors, or therapists (and clients!) of any stripe truly interested in learning to live and help others live with a free and enthusiastic CORE. If you won't probe who you are, you have no business asking others to change, release, and move into who they are.

*Mywhy* tells me health or healing comes from the restoration of the flow of energy through the body. Something or someone has caused most of us to stop that flow, and we'll find health when we remember how to resume it. I'm supported in this belief by many health models:

- the chakra system from India

- the Oriental medicine model of qi/ki/chi flowing through meridians

- the craniosacral model of cerebrospinal fluid movement through the spinal column
- the chiropractic system of osseous spinal freedom
- the osteopathic system of fascial manipulation
- the manual lymphatic drainage system which moves stagnant lymph
- the electromagnetic system of the body, which is finally being scientifically measured and given credence

and most specifically:

- the Ida Rolf method of structural integration (Rolfing) in which I trained, as well as other systems that in their way challenge us to reclaim the flow of energy.

No matter what system of health and healing we examine, we find the restoration of energetic circulation to be a major component. And that's where currently practiced medicine from our doctors too often fails us. It supplements deficiencies with drugs which teach the body to become dependent and forget how to function on its own. It often further dampens, slows, or stops energy to relieve symptoms. Too often this doesn't work. While they endeavor to improve health, too often medical practitioners stop energetic flow. Imagine taking your car to a mechanic when the "check engine" light comes on…he won't just put a piece of black tape over that light! Yet, too often, that's how medicine views "helping" patients, by masking their symptoms.

This book aims to help you find, then live and work from, your core space: mental, emotional, physical, energetic. Call it a self-help book for those who help others. I hope to help you enhance your clients' vitality, which should be a goal of any good therapy. But foremost, I want to prod you to more fully challenge self to find core before you ask others to energize their cores, freely and in touch with body and emotions. Too many of us try to shorten, hide, or make a smaller target with one or more pieces of our body to protect old emotional energy cysts. It's my goal to ask you to consider stretching, softening, and returning energy to your tight and tied places so you can feel physically and emotionally freer, and learn to *stay* that way.

Thereby you earn the right to challenge others to look at and release their bodymindcore blocks. I use the term "bodymindcore" because whether one addresses body or mind, both are intertwined in and emanating from the core at all times.

I call my work CORE (Coax Order and Restore Energy) Fascial Release because I'm more and more intrigued with finding, and helping clients find, this CORE space, through the tissues, but also through the emotions. I trained many years ago in Structural Integration and have evolved my interpretation of this work, while incorporating many other techniques over those years. While CORE Fascial Release is primarily about helping clients learn to recognize, pinpoint, challenge, and release physical or fascial tension or trauma, the longer I work the more aware I become that one can't merely work "on" a body: one must address the entire bodymindcore.

My intention as a bodyworker is to apply *moving* pressure to a particular physical static space in order to release stored trauma from connective tissue, which we'll discuss at greater length in Chapter 4 when we talk about stretching. During this work I'm consistently mindful that much physical holding through the connective tissue has an emotional rooting that must also be acknowledged. The emotional issues truly are embedded in the physical tissues. As I coax release from clients, I therefore encourage them to release their held patterns, be they mental, physical, emotional, or energetic of whatever sort. Static energy must be moved!

I hope to challenge you as a therapist to allow your intuition to become one of your favorite tools. Too many of us therapists ignore or disbelieve our intuition, even if we think we're honoring it. We find it hard to step outside our model and look at the larger picture— the energetic health of the client. I hope to convince you that you'll become even better at your work when you move beyond merely touching to sensing what's going on in the client's bodymindcore as you work. Most really good practitioners I know, and probably most you know, already feel and experience much of what I talk about in this book.

Read and experiment with this book for yourself; try the stretches, cues, and challenges you find here. The *Remember* feature at the end of chapters is meant to recap major points of the chapter, challenge you to look at yourself, and provide conversation starters with your clients that can help them begin to dissolve their blocks. I've given each chapter a general *All Purpose Cue*: any time you hope to free a physical area described, this cue would be appropriate to give nearly any client, verbatim, as the quotation marks imply. I've divided *Client Challenges* into *Easy, Medium, Difficult, Intriguing,* and *Imagine.* While *Easy* to *Difficult* ideas are for clients, *Intriguing* and *Imagine* may stretch the therapist.

Challenge yourself to first soften your own core. If you won't do the work for yourself, you have no business doing the work *to* others. Health is client centered, but healing is relationship driven, so a health facilitator creates a relationship with their client through good communication. The health facilitator takes the client to the brink of their fear or pain, then motivates them to bridge the gap to the freedom on the other side of the pain. He or she takes them past the question "Why (do)?" into the more productive question "Why not try (to do)?" He or she can't do this without first asking the same of self.

Other than 25 years of successful practice, why do I have credibility? A severe accident in 1987, shortly after Rolf certification, badly damaged my spine; nerves were crushed and doctors weren't sure how much function I'd retrieve or even if I'd walk. The journey back from that deeply traumatized body (neither quick nor easy) has taught me much of what I want to share here. A large part of that sharing is this: Whether dealing with physical, mental, or emotional pain or blockage, it's important to reach inside and examine, soften, and process to eliminate pains and fears.

Why soften? I think of softening as a step on the way to dissolving. If we're serious about making changes in those patterns that no longer serve, we must acknowledge and soften to dissolve and release. Many of us resist softening and try to hold ever tighter; creating brittleness and fragility—the opposite of softening, but also the opposite of strength. I suggest you encourage clients to allow their body's weaknesses to betray them and tell them what they need instead of allowing them to strengthen everything around the problem to try to pretend nothing's wrong.

This book elaborates on my earlier book for clients: *Meet Your Body: CORE Bodywork and Rolfing Tools to Release Bodymindcore Trauma* (Karrasch 2009). *Meet Your Body* asked the client to get up and *do* something: to begin moving and stretching the body machinery through a system that pays attention to the stuck or rusty "hinges" of the body, and to pull them farther away from each other. It's a book you may want to recommend to clients who are interested in taking charge of their healing. I'll recap this first book briefly in Chapter 2. *Freeing Emotions and Energy Through Myofascial Release* challenges the practitioner to go a step further and consider how suppression of *emotions* has created bodymindcore blocks on that central energetic channel of being, that essence around which life and world are organized. These frozen old traumas need to be stretched and released to help us all free *physical* pain and restore energetic flow. This book encourages a deep line of physioemotional or somatopsychic stretching awareness that calls us to also dislodge embedded thought patterns that still cripple or hinder many of us.

We'll endeavor to learn to simultaneously stretch two, three, or more places out of the holding patterns we consider our normal state. While we'll still stretch tissues, we'll ask the emotional issues in the physical tissues to let go as well, as we seek restored energetic function and flow. I intend to help you discover what you're trying to show clients about themselves, by showing you in yourself. I'm going to suggest a new vocabulary of directions, such as *downlong* or *upback*, that I encourage you to expand for yourself, signifying how to stretch tissues in several directions at once.

In today's world we're overstressed and overworked and have forgotten or never learned how to use foundational muscles to operate our body machinery smoothly. We've dug in our heels, hidden our hearts, and/or tied our guts in knots to get ahead. Let's decide to make changes.

I'm asking us to consider, then spread, a profound idea, new to some: that we're each in charge of our own health and healing, both physical and emotional. Though when you're sick and you look to others for help, why not first turn to your own inner knowing? When clients trust us, can we reflect their innate knowledge to them? Can we more fearlessly choose to open, stretch, and admit the tension we carry as a result of past fear patterns and injuries (physical, mental, emotional, chemical, electrical, energetic, or otherwise; invited or forced upon us)? Can we soften these fear patterns and replace them with a new and enthusiastic energy for who we are and where we're going—to health and happiness? Can we do this for us and our clients?

This book challenges you to restore physical, energetic, and emotional health by changing posture, and to add this commonsense model into your personal toolbox to become a more effective therapist. The sixth and seventh chapters deal directly with an Ida Rolf suggestion that we learn to live with the head up and waist back. Other chapters add pieces to a postural/emotional formula I've developed to help students and clients learn to open their core. There's no one universal formula or protocol for every individual! Each of us has our own DNA and life path as well as physical, mental, and emotional history. The order of chapters/centers I've chosen doesn't reflect the best way into *every body*; merely a good way in to most. One could easily start at toes or head and work straight through; any combination might have merit. Follow each body's directions.

Each chapter aims to teach our clients to help themselves stand taller, feel more confident, and move into the world more happily. If you practice the physical instructions first and let yourself feel the feelings *you've* held inside, you'll be better able to coax similar release of feelings, and trauma, from your clients.

To postural and emotional ideas, I've also added ancient Eastern spiritual and medical commonsense wisdom—primarily the chakra system from India. I've discussed what and where chakras are, how they relate to physical and emotional conditions, and the fears that clog them. I hope to challenge you to use chakra awareness to create length in the spine. If this system is too foreign or unscientific for you, simply think of body centers, hinges, or segments. I hope you'll ask yourself, before you ask your clients, which energy center holds its breath most strongly in this body, and which leads the body through life? In fear, or in joy? Which centers are too close? Which don't talk to each other? Where's energy tied up, and where's it too free? My world really is this simple: If we can create space between groin, gut, heart, and head, we're already healing.

We'll contrast chakras with classical Oriental medicine (not TCM [Traditional Chinese Medicine], which is a later and westernized form of Oriental medicine), which teaches that illness comes when our personal energy loses touch with the energy of the larger world. Symptoms are seen as the body's attempt to cure its own illness. When we lose this energy exchange, we slow down and accumulate *matters* and turn them into *matter*. Oriental medicine employs herbs as well as acupuncture, acupressure, or shiatsu techniques to free energy blockages up and down transmission lines called *meridians* (similar to chakra *nadis*). The healer works to personally feel the client's concerns—spoken or unspoken. Too many of us try to understand our clients' problems through the filter of *our* past. We get in our own way.

We'll talk about organs and glands, which perform amazing service by putting the appropriate chemicals into the system at the correct time and place. I'm most intrigued with helping us all soothe and manage our "fight or flight" *adrenal* system, and lift it up/off the kidneys, which Oriental medicine sees as the bringer of health.

I enjoy the metaphysics of the body, but I'm also interested in the physics, so each chapter on a specific body segment will be grounded by one of my favorite CORE Fascial Release techniques for freeing that particular area. I believe if you explore these techniques, *carefully*, you'll become a better body therapist. I can't teach you good deep tissue work through a book, but this book can stimulate you to explore deep work if you'll respect the power of these techniques and use them wisely. Such techniques won't work every time, but will hopefully give you permission to identify and trace lines of holding in your clients' bodies, as you feel such in your own. I'll add movement and awareness cues to help you, and clients, realize how we perpetuate our own holding patterns. We'll leave you with some "whys," but hopefully also give you some new "hows."

You'll also notice most illustrations in this book aren't extremely technical; there are no photos of techniques and most pictures are simple line drawings. This is done on purpose. I want to *suggest* stretches and muscles for you to consider. There are plenty of good anatomical drawings and slides already; my intention is to get you thinking of bodies and emotions more intuitively, as the illustrations do.

So I hope to introduce you to a new world—your own energetic bodymindcore—and to challenge you to open, soften, and restore the essence of who you are, before you interfere or interface with the worlds of others. I invite you to meet your body, your emotions, and your CORE experience.

It was the early physician Paracelsus who first suggested that the only dis-ease is congestion. The more we can learn to allow ourselves to admit to and soften all the congestion in our lives, then release that congestion and allow circulation through our bodymindcores, the healthier we as individuals and as a society become. My intention for this book: to make you a healthier and happier practitioner contributing healing to a healthier and happier society. If this still feels like, sounds like, or makes common sense to you, read on...

# MEET YOUR BODY

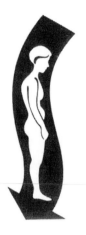 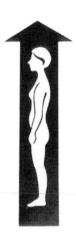

## A REVIEW

*Learn to create and find stretches that move each of
the body's many hinges away from each other to
enhance overall body function and feeling.*

A few years ago I created a book to give clients ideas and techniques to help them reclaim freedom in their own bodies. *Meet Your Body* (Karrasch 2009) has been a valuable tool to many; bodywork students as well as clients have found its ideas sound and workable. I continue hearing good reports about how working with this simple book has created positive changes for many, so I feel it would be useful to recap briefly its major premises before sharing what comes after it.

The book developed because of an injury I sustained to my right knee years back. Practitioner friends on both sides of the Atlantic worked to help me reclaim that knee with little success; finally I decided the old saying, "Physician, heal thyself," made sense and began to work on my own. I began trying to lift my weight through my big toes; particularly on the foot with the damaged knee. Immediately, simply by lifting into the big toe, that right knee and hip ached dramatically.

That was the insight moment: We must begin with the body's foundation and release or "oil" each of the hinges up through the body, first in ourselves and then in our clients. I had to begin retraining that hinge in my big toe to work by holding onto a counter or railing and using my arms to lift myself into my toe and through its traumatized hinge. Eventually I was able to stand on the right leg and lift myself through the toe unassisted; today my knee problem is gone.

## THIRTEEN MAJOR HINGES

This personal experience set me thinking about the various hinges of the body, and I chose to focus on 13 major hinges, or sets of hinges. I assigned specific exercises or stretches to each hinge so as to help clients "oil" or release them all. Obviously there are more than 13 body hinges; the spinal segments alone make 25 or 26 hinges, and fingers and toes have another 28. Clearly I treat some of these groups as a unit.

Partly because of my own body's experience and partly because of common sense, I chose to begin at and work up from the big toe hinge to encourage movement through a horizontal toe hinge, more than allowing the body weight to rise into the outer, smaller toes. I find that working to horizontalize and strengthen this big toe hinge creates amazing results for many health challenges. I've had clients tell me they've been able to cure plantar fasciitis, improve their varicose veins, keep back pain under control, and even lose weight just by learning to plant their feet straight ahead and rise and fall, slowly, through this big toe hinge. If you as a practitioner receive nothing else from this book, I hope you'll begin to be more aware of the horizontality of clients' toe and ankle hinges—no matter what particular therapy you practice.

Encourage clients to stand with feet on straight and sitting bone width apart, then rise slowly into the big toes—not to the outer ones! Whenever they have a moment, they can lift and sink, slowly, three or four times. I believe they'll begin to feel steadier, yet looser in their feet, and I believe they'll also begin to circulate energy through their legs and even the entire body more fully. This is foundational! The more energy we can find in our big toes, the healthier our body can become. I give this simple exercise to many clients.

Next I moved to the ankle hinge. If the big toe is properly lifting the foot, the ankle is already involved in efficient movement, but for too many of us neither toe or ankle work properly. Imagine the ankle is like a car axle: As we observe too many people we see high inner arches which denote a crooked ankle axle, with its outer wheel driving in the ditch. Flat feet see that hinge collapsing toward a center line. The more we can align the ankle and footbed properly to keep a horizontal ankle hinge while weight stays in a horizontal big toe hinge, the more the entire body above will be supported, and support the person. I suggest using simple squats while tracking feet straight ahead to strengthen and level the ankle hinge.

When toes and ankles hinge properly and we move to the knees, things get tricky. The knees are designed to be our best shock absorber, yet too many of us protect them by shuffling through life. If we add energy to our toes and ankles *as* we soften the tension in hips, knees can come to life and serve as the shock absorbers they're meant to be. Squats and knee bends are tremendously important to creating healthy knees, as is proper tracking, or placing toes, feet, knees, and hips in alignment from side to side before standing or stepping. I also suggest using steps as a piece of exercise equipment instead of a challenge to be avoided. Attention to knees and their alignment, and remembering to work them instead of favoring them, can absolutely change your client's world.

The hip presents a new hinge: a ball and socket joint. When some of the ligaments holding this ball into the socket get too tight, especially involving lumbosacral (LS) and sacroiliac (SI) junctions and low back hinges, we begin to have problems. Tight muscles follow; the feet turn out again, the low back begins to hurt, and the entire being suffers. Again, by practicing correct posture and tracking below the hips, we're beginning to allow clients to soften and allow movement through the hips.

My favorite stretch for the hips is called the Z position: sitting on the floor with both feet off to one side and both knees sinking toward the floor. Thus the legs form a zigzag line. Sit in this posture and experiment with making small quarter circles with your upper body—lift and circle (Figure 2.1). When you find the quarter circle that doesn't move smoothly (tension in your thigh? Back?), continue to try to work through that pain or tension, stretching and breathing. The longer you work in this position, the more your higher sitting bone will settle into the floor. As it does, you're beginning to unwind hip hinges even farther. I give this awareness to many clients with knee, hip, and low back issues.

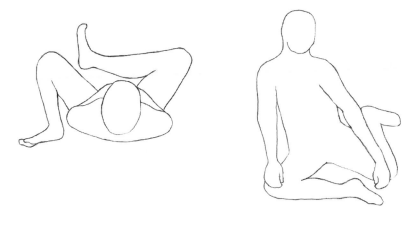

Figure 2.1 Z position

*Seen from above and from the side, the legs create a Z pattern in this stretch. Remember to put movement through the torso.*

## CREATING LENGTH BETWEEN THOSE HINGES

While writing *Meet Your Body* and thinking about hinges, the final challenge that presented itself to me was to create space between any two or more hinges as one stretched. Nowhere is this concept more evident to me than in the area between hip hinges and the low back or lumbosacral (LS) hinge. The LS junction is already a weak, tight, and anterior place on too many of us. By using the Z position exercise which asks you to sink the sitting bone down and lift the spine up *while* asking the low back to pull back, we're beginning to experiment with involving LS, SI, and low back hinges in stretching away from each other. This pulling various landmarks away from each other will be critical in this book, and we'll discuss it more in Chapter 4.

We can further teach clients to stretch this low back hinge by simple forward bends—allowing the body to roll forward as if the head and hands want to touch the floor, but working to find each spinal segment on the way down. Once they've reached the end of the forward bend, if they lift that lowest back hinge toward the ceiling and stack each hinge on the one below as they come up, they're further encouraging the low back hinge(s) to open.

This stretch also moves us right up into the stomach hinge...as we roll our segments back up, we'll exercise each of the 25 spinal hinges, not just the lumbosacral and stomach hinges. In general, my world and my advice to clients has become this simple: keep the waist back, no matter what activity you pursue, and you'll begin to learn to stretch and tone the stomach hinge.

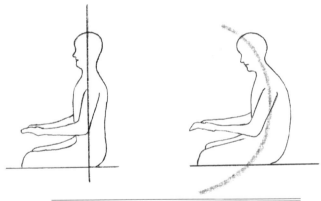

Figure 2.2 Heart in straight and slump posture

*Think of the physical and emotional reasons we close the heart area.*

The heart is the hinge I originally unwound for myself. I believe many of us have found a way to allow our heart area to shorten and tighten for various reasons that cut off both the flow of physical circulation and the emotional energy surrounding the heart (Figure 2.2). By encouraging clients to simply sit and stand tall, leading with the heart, they can make changes in physical and emotional well-being. We'll see the importance of the heart, which Oriental medicine sees as the Emperor of the entire body.

I see the arm hinge(s) and the shoulder hinge as separate entities. When I look at an arm and see it function well above the head or down to the ground, it occurs to me that this hinge can originate as low as L5 with lower latissimus fibers, but can also originate as high as C1 trapezius fibers, depending on the function required (Figure 2.3). Any movement that encourages clients to find a new range of motion from the arms—circling, swimming, lifting—begins to reset and stretch the arm hinge in any of the many directions it's able to achieve.

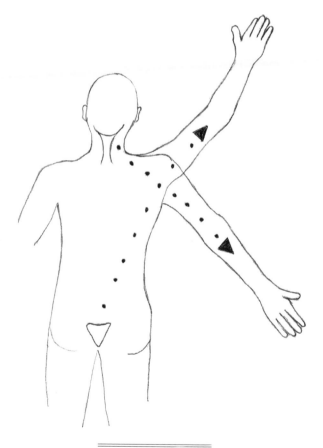

Figure 2.3 Arm hinge

*The arm hinge can be as high as C1, as low as L5, or anywhere in between, depending on the arm's function and direction.*

The shoulder, like the hip joint, is nearer a ball and socket than the other hinges. I believe we've lost much of the use of our "front legs" and think clients could benefit from letting their shoulders bear weight: doing four-legged animal walks and exercises, as well as swinging from trees, doorways, counters, or desks. I won't recap elbows, wrists, and fingers beyond suggesting that again, if we see them as front leg hinges and treat them similarly to the back leg hinges that correspond, we can make useful changes in a body's abilities and functions. Does a giraffe walk lightly in the big toes of the front legs, or in the heels? Does the bear lumber heavily in its back legs, or is it light on its feet? Does a reptile crawl on its belly, propelled by elbows? As we've become upright animals, we've lost the ability to allow our spines to be suspended from our shoulders. Some of our stretches will encourage this new/old way of thinking. We truly need to foster an ability to enhance both the range of motion and the weight-bearing ability this shoulder joint will allow if we're to help clients keep it useful.

My final hinge is the head… I imagine a four-part screen that's been collapsed too tightly at its three hinges, causing a head to pitch forward and shorten. When we teach clients to simply lift their head up and back, they begin to lengthen and unfold this screen (Figure 2.4). As a result, they've lengthened their body from head to toe. Their head is pulled up and out of their body instead of being jammed down into it.

## MEET YOUR BODY

*Meet Your Body*'s message: Learn to create and find stretches that move each of the body's many hinges away from each other to enhance overall body function and feeling. As you stretch/oil each hinge and pull it away from its neighbors, freedom follows. I'm interested in teaching you to teach your clients to find the muscle or area that feels fearful, angry, shamed, or stuck for whatever reason; then to encourage smaller and more subtle stretches and twists out of its pattern. This new book wants to take my client book a step farther: to teach you to coax your clients to now open both the physical tissues and the emotional issues that may be causing the physical problems. Let's challenge self and clients to find that "central channel" core line, and learn to stretch both it and all the hinges found along it.

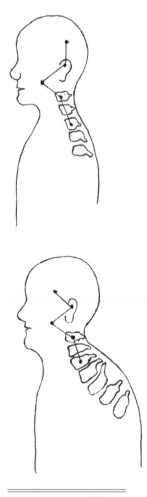

**Figure 2.4 Head hinge**
*See the head hinge as encompassing three pivot points:*
*Can you create length between these points?*

Let's add wisdom from my colleague, shiatsu practitioner Bev Breeze, who's been a tremendous help in planning this book. She gives therapists a great admonition; if her comment feels false or wrong to you, consider examining self more deeply or changing professions. Bev says, "I go in and ask the client to come out and meet me. Also in that meeting, I have to come out and meet myself, then keep going." Bev also asks:

*Do you consider how you "touch"? Do you receive information from the way you touch, or do you merely "do the job"? There's a lot going on if you care to listen and there's a lot you can affect if you work on yourself. Whatever work you do on yourself, whether it be bodywork or mind work, it will ultimately affect the quality of your touch. If you're healthy, strong, and vital, so will your touch be. Free your body and mind as much as possible...in shiatsu we work with "empty mind."*

This book challenges you to do your personal work to make you more available to your clients for your professional work. When you stretch your own core, you're able to help them stretch theirs. So, let's go!

CHAPTER
3

# THE CRUCIAL SPOT

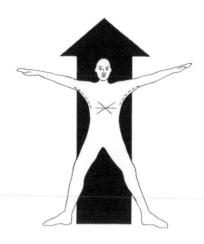

## THE FORT OF SELF—DEFEAT, OR WORTH?

*Lack of self-worth makes one tighten and hold their breath.*

First and foremost, I'm interested in getting myself, my clients, and you to breathe! Life would be so much happier if we'd simply put a little breath energy into it. Breath is free and not that hard; yet many of us hold our breath precisely to keep life at bay.

In my quarter century as a professional bodyworker, with basic and advanced certification in Structural Integration or Rolfing, I've studied and explored many techniques over these years of evolving my CORE Fascial Release Bodywork. I'm convinced the first and most lasting key to good health is learning to take in and let go of deep and cleansing breath on a regular basis. For me, the *only* dis-ease is the slowdown of energy, and too many of us slow down our energy by choosing to hold our breath. In Chapter 1, I asked which part of your body leads you. Which holds its breath? The answer to that second question may be that *all* your body holds its breath.

I often ponder sayings about breath, or lack of it: "She took my breath away." "His anger sucked the air out of the room." "That fall knocked the wind out of my sails." "The air was heavy in that place." Each of these sayings denotes a reason or stimulus that taught us to hold our breath, not move it. We do find positive phrases: "I heaved a sigh of relief." "She's a breath of fresh air." Which phrases make you happy and relaxed?

What takes our breath away? We do! Too often we respond to a stimulus from the world outside ourselves by stopping our breath. We seem to believe that holding our breath protects us by blocking the message or stimulus that's coming at us. While holding our breath may seem to keep problems at arm's length, we simply shorten our life and inhibit our activities by doing so.

Albert Einstein is reputed to have suggested the question he'd most like to answer was: Is the universe friendly? His superior reasoning abilities concluded that, indeed, we live in a friendly universe. He was able to act as if this was true. How well do you do that?

Consider: We may hold and apply an unresolved seed belief that the world is unfriendly, and remain anchored in that thought: We fear the future with dread. Like Job in the Bible, the thing we fear comes upon us and takes our breath away. We fear the present and the choice to move through it, so strive to shrink and be less visible. We hold our breath to take up less space and focus possible negative attention away from ourselves. We try to hold our breath until "it" goes away, or perhaps instead we go as hard and fast as we can to outrun our fears.

Even worse, we get anchored in the past: "Since I still have a sore spot (or the ghost of one) where that old hurt lives, I don't breathe into it." "When I visit stuck memories, I hurt. I don't want to hurt, so I won't breathe." Common knowledge now asks patients to get up more quickly after surgery to prevent painful restrictions caused by disuse; common sense tells us the way to get through any difficult task or pain is to plunge in and move. If it hurts either mentally or physically every time you breathe, how can you learn to acknowledge and push through that pain barrier to the freedom that lives beyond that old unsatisfied pain signal?

As we hold our breath, we starve our core. Without breath, we can't deliver oxygen to the lungs; they can't clean blood returning to be oxygenated; the heart can't pump revitalized blood. We become tired, lethargic, and ill simply because we don't breathe deeply.

How do you react when I suggest you "bring breath into" one of your physical trouble spots? How would your clients react? What if that spot's in the hip, or ankle? Don't the lungs take in and let out air? Why would I say "Bring breath into the hip"? I'm finding amazing results by encouraging a client to find breath in their shoulders while I work in their stomach or pelvis or even leg area—releases are much stronger and longer lasting. I find that if I explain to my clients what I'm doing, and why, and how they can work with me, we accomplish much more in our sessions. You may already realize how helpful breath images can be to clients, but how do we make it more real for more of them?

I ask clients to imagine their entire body is a balloon with a smaller balloon inside, which we'll label "lungs." If they inflate the inner lung balloon, won't the body balloon have to expand too? (See Figure 3.1.) As it expands, if they restrict parts of the outer balloon to redirect that air displacement, can't they direct air to the top, bottom, or middle of the bigger balloon, the body? I believe they can. If you can redirect your air, can't you direct it toward the traumatized and stuck parts of your bodymindcore?

The movie title *Waiting to Exhale* reminds me how most of us go through life holding our breath. If we'd just exhale deeply and satisfyingly, suddenly the dam might be broken and we'd get back to the business of vitality. If there's little breath, are we truly alive? And if we can't get our breath, shouldn't we be sorting our life to see what's taking our breath away? By the way, as you read, have you taken a breath lately?

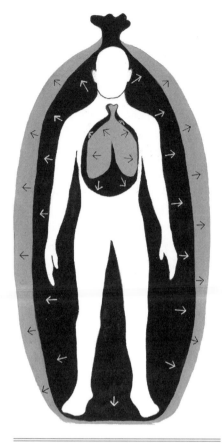

Figure 3.1 Double balloon in a balloon

*Imagine the lungs are a small balloon and the body is a large one…as the smaller balloon expands, won't it expand the outer balloon also?*

## NO BREATH, NO SPIRIT

Consider fibromyalgia. Most of us have dealt with this currently widespread and little understood condition, and doctors are unsure exactly what causes it or how to treat effectively. A fibromyalgia sufferer hurts—deeply, vividly. *Any* touch can be very painful. One key symptom is bilateral sore and tender points—both sides of the body experience pain the same way. Sufferers, more often women, have trouble getting deep sleep. Many times they're achievers who power through the pain until they can get home and collapse. Reducing stress, getting restful sleep, paying attention to diet, getting massage, and finding useful medication all may help alleviate their pain.

I believe fibromyalgia is simply a physical manifestation of "Something knocked the wind out of me and I can't get my breath back." While there's undoubtedly a chemical change in the body with this condition, it's triggered by this lack of breath. Fibromyalgia sufferers have usually experienced a deep physical, emotional, or chemical trauma shortly before the condition began—an assault to the CORE from their environment. So far every fibromyalgia client with whom I've worked has validated this observation for me. Their chemistry changed after they stopped exchanging air with the universe.

If you ponder the idea that sufferers had the wind knocked out of their sails you'll realize that by this definition nearly all of us are potentially fibromyalgiac. People who suffer most deeply seem to have not yet found a way to process and release trauma. Perhaps they were already wound more tightly or fearfully, or possibly their trauma was so quick and profound it totally caught them by surprise. Somehow, they're stuck. They need to find their breath mechanism's "reset" button, push through the blockage, and get on with their lives. I'm often able to help fibro sufferers release pain, just by helping them remember how to relax and breathe deeply.

I tell clients if they'd just drink more water, stretch, and learn to breathe correctly, they'd probably never need to see me again. I do believe health is that simple, and I'm particularly interested in trying to get clients to remember that breath is free and should be easy. Too many of us make breathing a difficult process.

## EASTERN WISDOM

Allow yourself to stop and think about a trauma you've absorbed recently—perhaps a physical sprain or strain; mental/emotional terror, shame, or other assault; or even chemical or energetic poisoning. As you remembered a trauma, did you feel the front of your body shrink slightly? Many of us do shorten our bodies as we react to trauma. If we focus on the area just below the heart while we relive a negative event or feeling, we may be aware of our fear causing us to close off and make a smaller target for the external threat. While trying to protect our core or essence, we starve it from breath and energy.

A *chakra* energy center is one of several specific points located along the spine and corresponding to a specific branch of our nerve network. Each of the seven major chakras is also one of my 13 *Meet Your Body* hinges. Most of us have some chakras and nerve patterns that are too open or active while others are too congested or inactive. We could all benefit from balance among and length between these energy centers. I sometimes think of the chakra system as an elevator; some of us only live on one floor, or never stop at certain floors as we travel from the head to the tail—if we travel at all.

Chakras originate in India; the Sanskrit word chakra translates as wheel or disc because energy seems to spin forth from a chakra, or to be stuck in it. While some people see these energies, I don't. Yet I believe the model is sound. The seven main chakras (Figure 3.2) as usually taught are these:

- *first* or *root* (between the anus and genitals)
- *second* or *sacral* (in the sex organs)
- *third* or *solar plexus* (the gut)
- *fourth* or *heart*
- *fifth* or *throat*
- *sixth* or *third eye* (just behind the eyes)
- *seventh* or *crown* (floating just above our head).

In a healthy body these centers work together to carry us on our journey toward awareness and vitality. As we work further with chakras, I'd suggest you begin to see three (too often) separate groups of chakras: 1–3, 4–6, and 7.

I see the following *phrases* as appropriate to these chakras:

- *root*: instinctively survive without fear
- *sacral*: responsibly create without shame
- *solar plexus*: honestly discern without judgment
- *heart*: enthusiastically quest without yearning

- *throat*: freely express without censorship

- *third eye*: rationally think without worry

- *crown*: consciously thrive without limits.

When any of these statements feels false, that portion of our body may be in trouble.

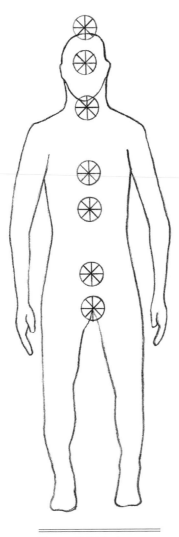

Figure 3.2 Chakra map

*The chakra system is made up of the seven traditional chakras.*

One could force a meeting of models by suggesting the Seven Deadly Sins and Seven Cardinal Virtues from medieval times correspond to these chakras. One might correlate:

- *root* with sloth or diligence
- *sacral* with lust or chastity
- *solar plexus* with anger or patience
- *heart* with envy or kindness
- *throat* with gluttony or temperance
- *third eye* with greed or charity
- *crown* with pride or humility.

When a chakra is focused on the positive virtue instead of the negative "sin," the entire being is energized; when we get the being alive in all chakras and focused on virtues instead of vices, sins, or shame, health ensues.

## THE BIGGEST STUCK SPOT

As we look at these traditional centers anchored up and down the spine, the first spot we'll consider isn't a chakra, but seems to me to be the *gateway* between the middle and low groups. If we have a constriction at this spot, our upper and lower body can't communicate, and we're strained throughout. Our elevator is stuck between floors, between the third and fourth chakras at the *diaphragm*. A truly gifted and graceful athlete, singer, or dancer may have resilience in their diaphragm; many have strength and tension instead. Can we help clients find resilience in this bodymindcore tightening? I think we can.

Imagine an umbrella-shaped muscle that forms the roof of the stomach and the floor of the heart (Figure 3.3). Imagine this umbrella is anchored at its edges to the lower ribs. Imagine the function of this umbrella is to push up and down, with the breath, in a way that moves air into and out of our lungs, expanding and contracting them. Too many of us have forgotten how to use this muscle and hold our breath.

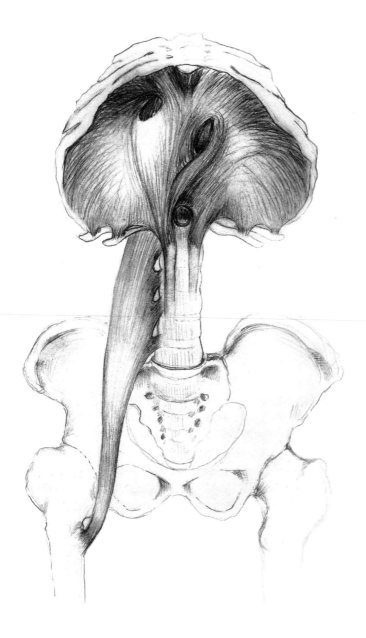

Figure 3.3 Psoas with diaphragm

*The diaphragm muscle can be thought of as the floor of the heart, the ceiling of the stomach, and the membrane that separates upper and lower chakras.*

Realize also how this diaphragm muscle has anchored just behind it, on the spine, the *aorta*, the main channel which delivers blood to the body. Openings or *hiatuses* in the umbrella allow the *vena cava* (which returns blood from the body to be cleaned and recirculated) and the *esophagus* (which allows food to descend through the area to the stomach) to penetrate the muscle. Common sense tells me when we hold our breath we tighten the diaphragm, and either choke these hiatuses and their tubes, or occasionally lose tone in them. We can't control the blood or food supply through this stuck place. We become congested, and ill.

For years I've taught that, at the center of our bodymindcore, we can visualize an hourglass. Actually, I perceive a series of hourglasses through the deep line of the body which correlate to these energetic chakras spaced up and down the spine. This diaphragm hourglass is my central and most important. I share this hourglass image with almost every new client within the first series of sessions, often their first session (Figure 3.4).

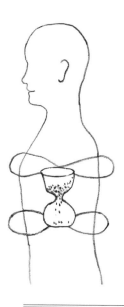

Figure 3.4 Hourglass

*Imagine the diaphragm (and its psoas connection) to be an hourglass:*
*When energy moves through, the upper and lower body communicate.*

In Oriental medicine the front of the spine, deep to superficial, has several pathways running right through this hourglass area (chakra model *nadis*). Visualize the diaphragm cords or crura descending to L2 or L3 on the front of the spine where they become nearly continuous with *anterior longitudinal ligament* fibers and with medial anterior fibers of *psoas* from T12 to L3. At the least, we're touching the deep essence of our client, as well as several deep Oriental channels and several more superficial meridians when we palpate the front of the spine. We're also working with the lower dantian or tanden: one of three centers defined in Oriental medicine (head, heart, gut), and the center of chi energy. As we move higher, toward the top of the diaphragm, we approach the second dantian center at the heart. This gate seems to be the connection of mind and body, and key to creating and maintaining health and energy flow. I find it's unfortunate that so many basic massage trainings ignore the stomach, which is key to moving energy.

Can you sense how many of us have a barrier between our upper bodies and lower ones where this diaphragm hourglass has tightened? Trauma/stress may have caused you, or someone you know, to hold their breath and clog this hourglass, cutting the body in two. In my practice nearly all clients are stuck here; it's usually the first place I touch each new client and many returning ones. Physical conditions we might develop as a result of our hourglass getting stuck include, but aren't limited to: emphysema and lung disorders, panic attacks and anxiety, hiatal hernia, acid reflux, and fibromyalgia.

It's my intention to tap clients' diaphragm hourglasses so the "sand" energy can pour through freely and appropriately again. I use bodywork tools and words to move this stuck energy. We've got to reset this core space to stay healthy. By paying attention to the form of our breath and exercise, and by learning to relax our minds as well, we can breathe ourselves to better health. With a bit of release work we can open a space on the *nadis* for communication between the lowest three and the highest three chakras.

## ACHIEVEMENT MODE

I talk to my clients frequently about "achievement mode." We may sit at the computer, stand at a counter, do household chores, talk with our spouse, work in a factory, drive our car, or even attend a yoga class for relaxation. Yet too many of us get into achievement mode at any task, and forget to relax and breathe. We've chosen to believe that, in order to complete whatever task has our attention, we hold our breath to power through it. As we hold our breath, the "sand" in our hourglass slows as the aorta, vena cava, and/or esophagus tighten. It doesn't register that we could achieve and breathe at the same time to reopen and maintain a "relaxed flow" or "relaxed process."

### CORE fascial release of upper psoas/diaphragm: My favorite

1. Client is supine. Locate the costal arch and let fingertips duplicate the angle of lower ribs, just below the 7–10 rib line, outside rectus abdominus.

2. Apply mild pressure in costal area until you feel you've hit a subtle, rubber wall. You'll both know, if you slow down. If you won't, you'll do damage.

3. Check in to client's pain or anxiety level (let them be in charge!), then tug tissue down to spine, down toward pubes, and medial toward linea alba, while client breathes. Careful! Pushing up/in could cause damage, so always tug tissue down. Ride the breath for three to four breaths.

4. Come out; see if breath has expanded from this touch.

5. You may choose to repeat the touch once or twice more.

6. Second touch: If you don't see expanded breath, put one fingertip on each side of xyphoid process and intend to tug tissue on the back side of sternum: up transversus thoracis tissue to sternohyoid muscle or through diaphragm to anterior longitudinal ligament, and therefore into shoulders, neck, and jaw. Client may feel a line of tension traveling to these areas. Always allow them to win the breath!

Too many of us believe it's hard to breathe because we haven't made learning to breathe fully and deeply a priority. What to do? If you're a practitioner with a shallow breath, try this awareness. If this isn't your problem, try this work with your problem-breather clients: "First, simply lie on the floor on your back, or even sit comfortably but with fairly straight posture, and focus on breathing in and out deeply and slowly. If you breathe in for a count of four or five, try to slow your breath to lengthen that count to six or eight. Take in the same amount of air if necessary, but inhale more slowly. After a particularly long in-breath, you may find the need to exhale in a rush; after a good out-breath, you may need a quick inhale. Without judging yourself for your lack of breath, intend to expand the time it takes you to breathe, then the *amount* of breath you're bringing into your systems."

Once you've experimented with longer breath, challenge clients a bit more: "Can you focus on bringing in more breath while staying in 'relaxed flow'? When working at your computer, or driving, or vacuuming, can you breathe at the same time? Notice your breath or the lack of it. Visualize this stuck hourglass at your diaphragm and teach yourself to allow more breath energy through it." As you become more familiar with tension in your own diaphragm, you'll be more able to help clients release their tension. Remember to start where your client is! If nothing moves and no time passes during their breath, praise them and encourage them to dig deeper.

## NOT GOOD ENOUGH

Why do we hurdle into achievement mode instead of enjoying a relaxed process? I agree with Louise Hay, author of *You Can Heal Your Life* (1984), who suggests most dis-ease is rooted in a lack of self-esteem. Many of us impose pressure on ourselves to do more and be better, and struggle to please others because we don't believe in our own worth. Lack of self-esteem is a disease many of us need to overcome, and most never quite do so.

In my final phase of Rolf training my work partner applied pressure under my ribs and just below the breastbone to release my diaphragm muscle. Since he wasn't finding his target, our teacher put his fingers near my breastbone for about one minute until something released, and moved on. Shortly after, I felt a great rush of freedom, followed by an intense emotional cleansing. The memory being freed was pre-verbal; the closest words were these: "I'm not good enough. I don't do enough. They don't want me here. I shouldn't have come."

My *soul* cried intensely for three hours. Each time I thought I was beginning to overcome the emotional pain, another wave washed over me and the crying started again. I left that session minus a large piece of the self-doubt that had tightly bound my core/essence since early in life. I've never been the same since that day. So when I write this foundational chapter I'm writing from definite personal experience and observation that lack of self-worth makes one tighten and hold one's breath.

I believe when you lie to yourself, your body shortens. I believe most of us have convinced ourselves we're not good enough—a lie— and have therefore shortened and tightened our CORE being. When we allow breath/circulation and feelings of self-worth to flow, we're on our way to health. When we find this freedom, or a part of it, we're able to help others find it.

# Remember

- Most of us are afraid of our pain, so try to ignore it or mask it. If we can face our pain, breathe, acknowledge its message, and stretch into and through it, we're on our way to releasing that which takes the wind out of our sails. When we don't face our pain we hold our breath, tighten our cores, stop our own flow of energy, and further our pain's hold on our well-being.

- When the hourglass between solar plexus and heart gets too tight (or loose) as a result of diaphragmatic imbalance, breathing problems, digestive problems, and circulatory problems may manifest in the body. As the diaphragm tightens, the hiatuses which allow blood and food to move through the body become irregular and disrupt the body's main supply lines. Upper and lower chakras can't communicate and we get stuck in specific body segments.

- Lack of self-esteem causes many of us to hold our breath. If we live in a world where we're not good enough, don't do enough, and can never change that pattern, we'll try to take up less space at the CORE or we'll try to achieve more and more externally to prove our worth—working ourselves to death.

## All purpose cue

"Work to learn to take deeper, longer, slower breaths; and remember to create opportunities when on task to find breath as well."

## Client challenge

### Difficult

I encourage clients and students to learn to breathe in slowly up to a count of 30, or even longer; then to quickly exhale and inhale before breathing out for a count of 30. As you repeat this cycle a few times, you've exchanged the oxygen-deficient air deep in your lungs, and created a healthier you. Don't worry if you can't reach 30; it's a goal, not a test.

### Imagine

Pay attention to the situations and people that "take your breath away": Can you alter these situations and people? Do you choose to avoid them, confront them, or find a new way of being that allows your breath to flow?

# CHAPTER 4

# NOW, DO SOMETHING!

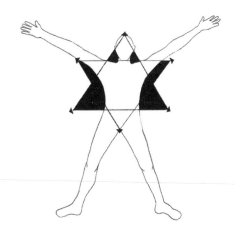

## THE BIG ONE—LOSE, OR USE?

*One who is unwilling to stretch and live outside their comfort zone becomes brittle, loses elasticity, and is prone to injury—mental, physical, and emotional.*

*Resilience, not strength, is the goal of my stretching or workout.*

Imagine an elastic or rubber band. If one holds the elastic by only one end, it's impossible to stretch. In order to achieve a stretch, we need two anchored ends moving farther apart—we have to stretch *from* something. If we want to create even more resistance, we not only stretch both ends of the band; we twist them at the same time. If we further put a foot or knee at the middle of the stretching elastic and pull it away, we've created yet one more direction in which we can stretch.

This idea is critical to my work: the more directions you can challenge your clients to stretch at once (when you're working with them, as well as when they stretch for themselves), the more they'll be able to soften and create resilience through the entire bodymindcore. Conversely, I find one who is unwilling to stretch and live outside their comfort zone becomes brittle, loses elasticity, and is prone to injury—mental, physical, and emotional.

## STRETCH THE CORE

*What* are we stretching? In addition to the muscles you normally think of, we create elasticity in the connective tissue, or *fascia*. Fascia is a continuous webwork; a tissue network that wraps muscles and muscle groups and connects every part of the body to every other part. Although originally observed hundreds of years ago, fascia was first made the basis for a healing model by Andrew Taylor Still, founder of the osteopathic technique.

Imagine millions of cobwebs running from every cell of your body to every other cell. In addition to connecting various segments of the body, fascia gives the organs and muscles support and structure and provides a communication system that connects all the body's tissues with all others.

If you imagine that every air bubble of a sponge is full of muscle tissue, the sponge is a bit like fascia—consistently offering structure and support to the muscles. Visualize cling wrap as it comes off the roll; if we're not careful it immediately glues to itself and we have to wet it to free it. Think of toffee or salt water taffy that's become hard and brittle; if we chew or massage it, the hardness becomes resilient and pliable again. Without work, it may be impossible to even remove it from the wrapper. We need to hydrate, clean, and free our body's connective tissue system, which also stores our energetic slowdown, emotional tensions, and physical reactions.

The longer I work with fascia, the more I'm convinced of its power. I continue experimenting with ways to open and stretch various body parts, and ways to move chakra centers away from each other, as I ask my connective tissue system—and my clients'—to regain pliability. For someone with such injury and abuse in their body, I'm quite flexible. Recently my first spinal X-rays in 18 years confirmed a very healthy spine and neck, considering the history of physical damage I carry in my body. My spine may be fused, but it's not inflexible or unhealthy.

Think of a new balloon that's never been inflated. The first thing most of us do before we attempt to get air into this new balloon is to stretch it. Without this tugging, it's going to be much more difficult to make this balloon accept air. The act of preparatory stretching creates resilience and adaptability to change. Our connective tissue, our bodies, our minds, our lungs, even our chakras and emotions, are like this balloon. Let's stretch them so that energy can again flow freely.

## SIMPLE, GOOD RULES

Let's make a few ground rules to help us teach clients to stretch more efficiently.

First: Breathe, always! Training ourselves to nourish our bodies with breath can change everything in our world for the better—including our minds.

Second: Use it or lose it. Too many of us stand, feel a weakness in our knee or leg or back, and choose to favor it and allow it to inhibit our movements. Wrong! It really is as simple as taking an extra moment to load ourselves correctly into our feet, level our pelvises, lengthen our spines, and move forward from an upright and efficient position instead of a forward-bending, trauma-favoring achievement posture. Choosing to move into and through pain, instead of bracing against it, gives us the opportunity to soften and work that pain free, physically and emotionally.

Third: When stretching (with breath), how much is enough? This is such a tricky question, because each of us must become our own authority! Though current research suggests 30 seconds may be an appropriate holding time, let me share what works for me. When I stretch, I take myself to the edge of the place where I wonder if I've stretched too deeply. Then I slow and relax. How do I know if I'm pushing too hard? I inhale—if

I can inhale fully, I'm stretching appropriately. If I can't get a full breath, I'm working myself too hard and need to back off, stretch less, and try the breath again. When I think I've found my optimal stretch, I hold for a "small stretch." It really is that simple—the more you remember to monitor how hard you work yourself and let yourself move through the stretch and breath simultaneously, the more good work you do. Too many clients want you to be their authority, but it's your responsibility to develop their responsibility.

Fourth: Static or moving stretch? New research actually suggests static stretches, where one goes to a limit and holds, are less effective and potentially more injury-producing than non-static, moving stretches. So, keep moving!

Fifth: As we divide the body into segments for the chapters of this book, challenge clients to stretch various segments or chakras farther away from each other. We'll talk more to this idea throughout the book, and conclude there are posturally four major points to keep open and long—groin, gut, heart, and head. Keep in mind that holding both ends of an elastic band will make it stretch much more effectively; it's the same in your body. Can you continue to find ways to stretch these four points away from each other? Our "client challenges" will encourage this deep line stretching, both for you and for your clients.

Sixth: How to stretch? How to teach stretches? Make it up. Can you experiment with different shapes? (See Figure 4.1.) Can you stretch your entire body in a straight line? Can you form your body into a forward or backward "C" curve? A teardrop? A "Y" or "Twisting X"? Can you also mildly swing and sway when you're stretching your body? Challenge clients to experiment. *Any* activity of daily living could bring a stretch to the entire system. We could even stretch as we sit to watch TV. Yet if we approach an activity in "achievement mode," we won't get the stretch *or* relaxation benefit from the activity. It's more important to dialog with the body instead of pushing it to its limits.

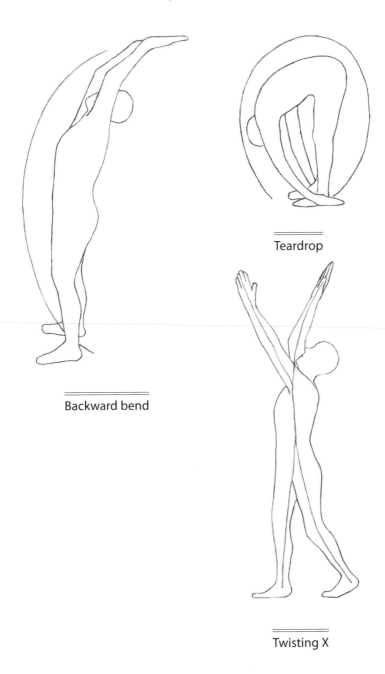

Teardrop

Backward bend

Twisting X

Figure 4.1 Stretches in design

*Can you invent stretches that challenge your body in several directions at once?*

And seventh: Let's create a new language around stretching, based on my elastic band. This is an ongoing creation: I'm merely suggesting a language of words that denote one, two, three, or more directions of stretch. Throughout this book I'll encourage you to stretch your head upback with feet floordown while knees stretch insideupback. If you break any of these words down, they'll hopefully make sense. For example, if you're lying on your back and I suggest bringing your stomach skyup, you know what I'm asking. In each chapter see if you can duplicate the directions I've suggested, or create your own.

Return to the elastic band and consider stretching two or more *chakras* away from each other at once. Generally, you won't go wrong creating stretches for self, and client, that ask feet and legs to stay downlong while head and neck or shoulders, arms, and hands reach upback. To add that third and fourth direction, what would happen if your stomach hinge moved back while your pelvic hinge moved down at the same time?

However you stretch, or teach stretches, encourage deep inhalation *into* the discomfort; hold, then *ex-press* and *ex-hale* the guards set at the borders of the pain. Ask clients to use that which is around them: stretch at the bus stop—stretch in the car seat while waiting for the stoplight to change—stretch in the mornings and evenings while brushing teeth—stretch by hanging from a doorway trim when moving through a door. When you stretch yourself firmly but safely you can teach your clients what they need.

I've lately come to another realization: Resilience, not strength, is the goal of my stretching or workout. Although I'd like to be strong at 80, I'd much rather be flexible and resilient then. I believe too much strength creates a tightness that ends up being weakness, brittleness, and fragility. I'd rather have a resilient CORE that operates safely and happily in its environment, takes in, processes, and discharges any pain, and freely moves from the inner to the outer world and back without holding on against pain or snapping due to tension.

## CORE fascial release: Rules for my work

1. Coax tissue, never force. Stay on the appropriate layer where client remains present. Respect the tissue and the person.

2. Watch the way they move or don't move. Listen to what they say or don't say.

3. If client is more comfortable clothed, can you allow them to remain clothed?

4. Keep moving, always, and keep your direction moving across tissue, not straight down into it. The deeper you want to work, the slower you go.

5. Ask for breath and movement from the client as you work. Are they still in their body, or have you tightened them further with too much, too fast, and too deep?

6. Communicate: What you're doing, why it could help, and how they can help create healing.

7. Challenge client to stretch energy from groin, gut, heart, and head in as many directions as possible.

8. Give client small assignments at the end of the session to prolong and deepen the change.

9. Withdraw/let go! Client has you for an allotted time. It's honest to leave them in charge.

# STRETCHING EMOTIONALLY

And if I stretch emotionally with the above rules, my world is an easier and happier place. Whatever comes at me intensely and causes me to shorten, hide, or make a smaller target, I try to stay with that emotional sensation and find a way to *soften* it: understand, process, and work through the feeling instead of allowing it to anchor in my physical tissues. I try to get bigger when my emotions tell me to shrink my connective tissues. The message is creating health and happiness, for me and my clients.

Another key: Whether our pain is emotional or physical, I suggest we've got to go below and beneath the current pain into and through older pain when we stretch. We must revisit deep and early hurts, even if we don't know what they are. We've got to feel our pain; look it in the eye, stretch, and breathe to release its power over us. It's simple; it's not easy. While we may not know what the pain is about, we've got to acknowledge it to release it.

When I work to release a client's tensions with touch or intention, I think in terms of layers: At layer one, the client feels they're being pampered…no challenge. At layer two, the client begins to register concern: "What's going on in me right now, and will I be all right if I move into and through this sensation?" At layer three, the client decides it's no longer safe to stay in the body while the therapist (the/rapist?) assaults it. Put another way: I'm interested in doing proximal release work in bodies, as deeply as I can, including release with my words. But sometimes a body tells us our proximal or deep work must be done on a distal or superficial layer. We've got to get better at reading client signals.

One of my mentors, Louis Schultz, anatomist and movement instructor at the Rolf Institute, and author of *The Endless Web: Fascial Anatomy and Physical Reality* (1996), used to suggest to us as students, and to his clients: "Now go home and *play* with this idea…" This is sound advice—*play* with creating more stretches in more directions, to acknowledge old pains, as deeply as you can, in yourself, and in your clients.

I suggest we pay attention to bodymindcores in a new way. Let's reshape our minds and feelings: dismantle outdated coping patterns, let go of old addictions, shake out collected traumas, allow energy to flow through us, and learn to feel praise and gratitude for our bodies as well as our emotions. I challenge us all to see our bodies as the vehicles that take our emotions out into the environment to enjoy, experience, and serve our greater world. Why can't we learn to maintain our bodies in a way that serves both our core and our environment? And how can we challenge others if we don't challenge ourselves?

Appropriate movement is purposeful, not forced; on purpose, not random; and self-directed, not externally driven. Appropriate movement comes from the CORE or deep line, not the sleeve or external muscles. It's lived, not achieved nor pinched off at the diaphragm, and fueled by appropriate breath. Life is meant to be lived in an expansive mode, not a contracted one. Stretch, don't shrink.

## Remember

- Think of an elastic band: the more directions one can stretch that elastic, the more resilient it becomes. Our bodymindcore's *connective tissue or fascia* behaves the same, so experiment with creating more and more directions to stretches. Imagine you can create length between spinal segments and between chakras. Visualize an internal elevator moving smoothly through all body segments.

- When stretching and breathing, be sure to take a *moving* stretch to the physical place where breath is challenged, not beyond. Keep in mind that strength isn't strength; flexibility or resilience is strength. Let's be flexible in the tissues *and* the emotions.

## All purpose cue

"Create a ritual: It may be as simple as morning and evening time with breath and stretching. Perhaps you'll learn to breathe every time a stop light interrupts you, or train yourself to stretch before you answer the phone. Create a pattern or habit that helps you learn to breathe and take up space more fully and more often. Train yourself to believe you could breathe, move freely, and get longer in every situation instead of shortening, tightening to protect yourself from all challenges, real or imagined."

## Client challenge

### EASY

Set an egg timer or "minute minder" for varying amounts of time. When the bell rings, check in to see how you're treating your body and emotions...are you open, relaxed, and stretched out? Are you tight, tired, on guard, and holding your breath? Can you allow yourself to find "relaxed" more often?

## MEDIUM

Consider your work space and posture…what can you change to make work more comfortable and friendly to your body?

## DIFFICULT

Think about a specific body part that bothers you often: Can you create a stretch that asks distant body parts to pull away from the painful area? For example, for a headache, can you try pulling the elbow out of the neck *while* pulling the opposite ear to its shoulder and out of the neck in the other direction (with breath)? For low back pain, can we pull the heel out of the back *while* pulling the leg long *while* the head stays long *while* the back stays back? Make up ways to involve your body in two, three, or even four directions of stretching at the same time.

## INTRIGUING

In coming chapters you'll see more new terms: upback, upover, earthdownlong, skyupbehind, and outlongback are directions you might soon find. Hopefully they'll make sense to you in relation to the idea of asking yourself to stretch in more directions at once.

## IMAGINE

I'm not sure how cursive writing or penmanship is taught in schools these days; as a child I practiced long lines of circles or loops, sharp up and down strokes, or the rolling hills of cursive "m"s. The repetition of these strokes gave us the opportunity to learn to make them even, clean, and uniform. Can you transfer this penmanship idea to stretches? Anywhere there's a shortening or tightening that causes a "stroke" to feel choppy, that stroke needs practice.

# CHAPTER 5

# TEST THE TOES

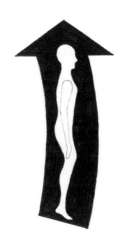

## AN AMAZING JOINT—CAN'T, OR WILL?

*How do my feet relate to the earth, and is this
the healthiest relationship I can create?*

*Fear is a basic shortener, tightener, traumatizer, and
killer; headlong enthusiasm is its counterpart.*

I've not heard others say this, but observation tells me that, physically, most of us are dying from the feet up. I watch people walk, and find the less spring in their step and the less toe and ankle hinge with each step, the unhealthier they are in the body above. They're shuffling toward a quicker death. If severely edemic clients could just learn to use ankle and toe hinges, their problems could be far less severe. Gravity makes toxicity settle to the bottom. In order to pump toxicity out of the body, we need healthy feet hinges. For too many of us, that pumping action just isn't happening. Why? Why does the old saying about "being set back on your heels" seem to take all our energy away? Conversely, why does someone who seems to be "really on their toes" feel complimented? I've tested many protocols or chapter orders for this book, but feet always come first after breath and stretches. They're critical to good health.

In 1987, just as I thought my life was going in a fantastic new direction and I'd found a new spring in my step, I fell out of the sky when my pilot friend ran out of gas in his small plane and made a forced landing. My body was devastated in that wreck, with a compression fracture of L1, neurosurgery, spinal fusion, and Harrington rods installed (and removed 18 months later). I've spent years regaining health. After chasing healing for so long, I've finally learned to ask myself some hard questions that seem to be restoring energy to my CORE and making me a better therapist and teacher. I'm going past the years-old plane wreck pain into even deeper and older emotional core pain and attendant physical holding. I'm integrating who I am and who I want to be by asking self, and now challenging students and clients to consider: How do my feet relate to the earth, and is this the healthiest relationship I can create?

As I watch people move forward, many seem to walk on eggshells or tiptoe through hot coals. Their relationship to the earth seems fearful. Others plod through life with no joy, no spring, no enthusiasm—defeated. It seems to me many of us are living with issues of safety—is this planet, and the next footstep on it, safe? Do we stay "on our guard" at every step? Are we de-feeted? Or are we among the few well grounded?

The feet, knees, and tip of the tail are governed by the first chakra, the root or base. The phrase I'd like us to ponder in regards to this chakra is "Instinctively survive without fear." Fear is a basic shortener, tightener, traumatizer, and killer; headlong enthusiasm is its counterpart. It makes sense to be aware and alert; it doesn't make sense to live in fear. Enthusiastic, but not hyper, vigilance is the cardinal virtue I associate with this chakra; sloth (defeat) is the vice. We'll talk to this first "survival" chakra again in the chapter focused on knees and loins.

Though chakra 1 is physically located at the base of the spine, between the anus and genitals, it governs toes to the top crest of the hipbone. It allows the body to circulate/eliminate energy and to remain grounded, yet dynamic, in its relationship to the ground. It sets the foundation for sure survival by protecting the body above. Though chakra systems often suggest the *adrenals* (the fight-or-flight glands) correlate to the third chakra (solar plexus/waist back), I believe the adrenals are critical to the feet and vice versa. Too many of us are in "fight" or "flight" mode, too often.

In classical Oriental medicine this first chakra area at the perineum could also be equated to the "Lower Burner" of three burners or processing body areas (lower eliminative, middle digestive, upper heart and kidney). The first chakra's physical location is the joining of the lower Conception Vessel (CV) and Governing Vessel (GV) meridians. Everything above is directly related to the CV/GV point at chakra 1, the basis of fear of survival or enthusiasm for life.

Let's examine for a moment the concept of yin and yang. Oriental medicine sees a universe where every action has a reaction and every condition has its partner. As the front of the body is more emotionally centered, it could be classified as yin; the back's physical energy is yang. Energetic/exterior usually signals yang; internal/quiet signals yin. I'm less interested in learning to diagnose deficiencies of either and more intrigued with accepting the idea that all things seek balance and need all aspects of their being to form the whole, and healing.

## YOUR OWN TWO FEET

Years ago Lucy was brought to me by her mother because her feet hurt all the time. After many medical consultations, Lucy and her mother heard two options: doctors could break and reset all the bones in her feet; or they could put her in a mental institution since the pain was all in her head. I guided Lucy through the ten sessions of Rolfing, and her pain diminished dramatically.

Somewhere near the end of her series, her mother confided in me one day: "Oh, I love being a mom—I wish I could have babies forever. Lucy's my last and I just couldn't let loose of her...I carried her everywhere for her first five years." Light bulb! Too often, we have trouble allowing our offspring to stand on their own two feet. Does this challenge you to think at all about early walkers or babies with a strange gait? Do we ever truly grow out of first walking patterns?

Many of us live with a certainty we'll never measure up, reinforced by elders who want us to "watch our step" as they guide us through life without turning loose to allow our growth. My maternal grandmother was soft spoken but formidable, and I never felt good enough for her. With her "not good enough" messages deeply embedded in me, I never felt truly safe or competent. I couldn't stand on my own feet or defend myself after accepting I was less-than; an old pattern I still work to remove.

I learned to accommodate her low expectations with self-limiting behavior. Through the lens of time, I see my plane crash experience, even though I wasn't at the controls, as a self-negation. My gut didn't trust my pilot, who'd already run out of gas and lost power on his landing approach when we arrived at our destination. I knew I shouldn't board his plane again. I didn't trust his will to live, but I thought my will to live was grounded and strong enough for both of us. At this time I'd freed myself from so much. I didn't expect bad things to happen to me.

That crash nearly ended my life. I remember hearing my grandmother's voice in the early hours at hospital (not physically there, or even alive), saying, "Well, you've gotten into a mess now, haven't you? I don't think you'll ever get over this." How could I have thought the earth wanted to lovingly nurture and support me? It/I actually wanted to hold me back, for my own good.

Why do we self-limit and stumble so badly? Do we do so in order to please or appease or seek favor from someone? Have we been stifled by someone? If so, who? Why do we accept their evaluation? Who or what do we think we're honoring by "watching our step"? Is this pattern still serving us? Can we renegotiate a better relationship to ourselves and the earth?

## AM I PLEASING THEM?

Ask yourself and your clients: "Whom do you still honor (but rarely succeed) by whatever self-limiting behaviors you've chosen? Who's still telling you to 'watch your step'? Who won't let you 'stand on your own two feet'? Are you trying to achieve standards you imagine your elders had or still have for you? How does this pattern make you relate to the earth—joyfully, fearfully, resignedly? What destructive behaviors are you still choosing? Are they life enhancing? Do they serve you? If not, why do you still give these unresolved negative thoughts power?" It's time to release old attitudes and behaviors to move forward, fearlessly, into the future. As you release, you'll better help clients.

When the Bible tells us to honor father and mother, I believe it suggests we honor their "being" or essence, while we discern the wisdom of their "doing" or behavior. It's not necessary to dishonor their being or doing by labeling them "wrong" as we free ourselves from well-intentioned but misguided parenting influences. I hope we all have come or can come to a point where we understand our parents did the best job they knew how to do in raising us, considering the tools they had in their kit. I honor my parents. Though perhaps they could have been more affirming, they guided me to here and now, and I'm grateful. I'm satisfied in my new under-standing and humbled by my own parenting trials.

It's my sense that as we let go of these stifling, outdated "watch your step" messages we become enthused instead of weary in our world. Not only can we find better balance in our bodies; I believe we'll tone, yet relax, that adrenal fight-or-flight mechanism which keeps us on guard. We'll change the energetic stagnation of our bodies through the loins and into the kidneys: edema, swelling, and varicose veins can release. We can even enhance a sluggish heart, circulatory, and lymphatic system if we stay relaxed, yet in our toes, believing the world isn't trying to knock us back on our heels.

Actress Maureen Stapleton obviously knew how to get out of the self-sabotage mode that others can train into us. When she joyfully bounded onstage to accept an Academy award in 1982 for her work as Best Supporting Actress in the film *Reds*, she thanked everybody she'd ever met in her entire life. Isn't that true? All the influences from the past have brought you to who you are today. If you can be grateful for not only who and where you are, but for *all* that brought you there, you're well on the way to the joy and groundedness you deserve.

## STAY ON YOUR TOES

So let's change how we *physically* create *emotional* happiness as we move through life. I've long been a believer in the idea of developing this "spring in the step" when we walk and stand. As a result of old injuries (maybe even a reason for them) I've realized I walk heavily in my heels with minimal toe or ankle hinges. As I've learned to spring through my feet, I've begun loosening my big toe and ankle hinges; my knees, my body, and my attitude feel better too. I hope you can find strength and resilience in your feet, and help your clients find it as well.

Return to the logo person at the beginning of this chapter: a body on its toes. Think of standing on a diving board. Come up onto your toes and add that toe-pushing spring that allows you to dive. I'd like us all to experiment with being on our toes in our lives. If we stand firmly in both feet and allow ourselves to rock slightly back and forth—into the heels, then into the toes—we discover what it could feel like to be slightly in front of ourselves and in our toes. Can you feel the muscles in the back of your legs coming alive? Do you see how easily you could bring this awareness to clients?

Do you put more weight in one foot and leg than the other? Most clients can notice some imbalance. It's possible that if one's weight goes more through the left side, they related more safely to their mother or feminine role model; if in the right side, the father figure was a safer model. Rolfer/psychologist Stacey Mills used to discuss this imbalance from side to side and found in her years of practice that it was often an accurate indicator of which parent was most present and/or absent. It's an interesting observation: Which inside of heel do you put into the ground most strongly? Does that coincide with the parent figure from whom you felt your main support?

Lately I've been challenging clients to make their footprints into mirror images of each other. I think the more our feet match each other as they connect to the ground, the healthier and happier we'll become. The next time you leave barefoot prints, examine them (Figure 5.1). Perhaps one arch is higher, or one foot looks shorter. Perhaps one foot points farther outside. As you try to match your feet with equal weight, what happens in your body? Do you feel tension in places above? Do your hips shift when your feet match?

Can you work to equalize your weight distribution? Can you evoke this discovery from your clients?

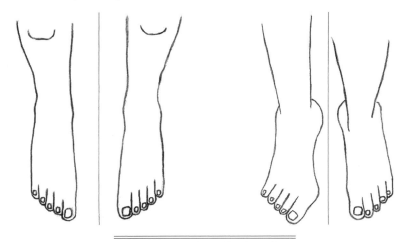

Figure 5.1 Good and bad tracking

*Correct foot tracking (L) and poor foot tracking (R) points out whether we know where we're going in life.*

"Focus on which parts of your feet carry the weight of your body. Massage your feet *and* body by shifting your weight from heels to toes and back, *while* you keep weight on the inside of your feet. Wake up! Then, experiment with other patterns. Send your weight into an outer crescent instead of an inner one; then a full circle or a figure 8, then a straight back and forth figure *while* you lift into the toes. Can you feel the leg muscles getting a new workout?" Train clients to stand *their* ground.

While it's important to be able to allow the weight to sink into the entire footbed, teach clients to put more weight into one spot behind their big toe and slightly inside, toward the center of their foot, to help energy rise through the body. In Oriental medicine this spot is called Bubbling Spring or Bubbling Well, and it grounds the Stomach, Liver, and Spleen meridians which travel up the front of the body as well as several deeper channels that travel near the front of the spine. I enjoy standing, shifting the weight of my body from point to point in my feet to massage this spring, and focusing on physical and mental sensations.

The muscle we're working to wake up with this shift into the toes travels deep in the back of the calf, behind the two bones of the leg and their interosseus membrane. Can you feel it? This deep muscle is the *tibialis posterior*, which simply means back of the tibia (bone) (Figure 5.2). As we create activity and resilience (not strength!) in the tibialis posterior, many things happen. Muscle action pumps blood back up the body, where it's cleaned and recirculated. We become physically more responsive—ready to move left, right, forward, or back more quickly. The deep line of the entire body begins to unwind and relax. We lose our "de-feeted" or on-guard attitude and move to enthusiastic readiness.

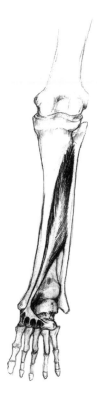

Figure 5.2 Tibialis posterior

*This muscle is just behind the interosseus membrane, between the tibia and fibula, and deep to the flexor muscles, gastrocnemius and soleus. Energy to it is critical to overall health and well-being.*

## CORE fascial release of legs:
## Tib post, flexors, and extensors—Spring in the step

1. Client supine if your fingers will tolerate the work; feet slightly off edge of table/couch.

2. Place fingertips on back of leg in the central channel of gastrocs; slowly intending to sink in and gently drag finger down toward heel.

3. Ask for client movement—toes and ankle up and down (horizontal hinge).

4. Intend to soften and release tibialis posterior and flexors through calf; then follow tib post out from under Achilles tendon and down behind inner maleolus. Next, find inner arch/flexor tendons and hold/lengthen with gentle pressure and horizontal ankle movement (little toe up towards face/big toe pulls foot down).

5. Front of leg, work up the outside of tibia bone through (first trip), then outside, tibialis anterior to release extensor muscles. Continue to ask for toe/ankle work.

6. You might choose to put a bit of work to the inside of tibia; here you nearly catch inner gastrocnemius, but also soften the meridian rising here. Work lightly! There's little muscle tissue here.

7. If client is too big, or your hands too fragile, turn client prone and use elbows, thumbs, or knuckles to soften the same lines on back of calf.

8. You might let client stand after one leg is released…usually they can tell a real difference!

Superficial to the tibialis posterior, yet deep in the back of the leg and all the way to the toes, we find the *flexor digitorum longus* and *flexor hallucis longus* muscles, which flex the foot or bring the toes down toward the ground. In front of the *interosseus* (between bone) membrane are their important partners, the *extensor digitorum longus* and *extensor hallucis longus*, or long extenders of the toes and big toe (Figure 5.3). Energy to these muscles is foundational.

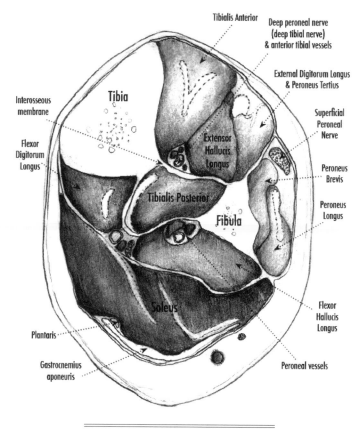

Figure 5.3 Cross section of right leg

*Note the interosseus membrane holding the bones together; the placement of the tib post and flexors, and the placement of the tib ant and extensors. These muscles connect the deep line of the leg to the toes.*

There's so much we can do for ourselves to open and energize the legs. Try these ideas; then share with clients when appropriate: "Lie down with your feet resting up on a chair. Can you simply pull your toe hinges farther away from your ankle hinges (downlong)? First point your toes long and as far away from your ankles as possible; then pull your toes toward your body (upfront) and stretch your *ankle* downlong. Can you then draw crescents with your toes *while* stretching your heels long and your toes up?" We're waking deep muscles, stretching front and inner meridians, and energizing all the chakras.

"As you stand and take a step forward, you probably already feel your legs are more alive. Experiment with walking with a spring in your step and using your toes to push off the ground (Figure 5.4). With each step, allow yourself to connect the ball first and your heel a bit (though not too heavily!). Allow the toe to push your foot up and into the next step. You may even wish to come up and down in your toes a few times before the first step, to 'oil your hinges.' Now, can you also allow your waist back, your head up, and sink your knees into your feet as you spring from your toes?"

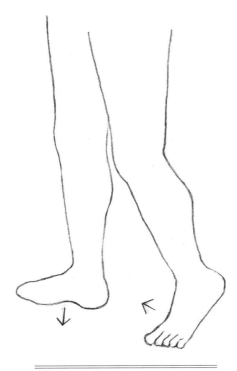

Figure 5.4 Walking with toe hinge

*Walking in an upright body with less weight in the heels allows deep muscles to activate and creates shock absorbency.*

Current research and shoe development suggest that barefoot running makes sense to our bodies, since it allows us to use all the muscles of the foot and leg to receive and absorb the shock of the earth, and spring off from it more fully. Isn't it common sense that the more we allow our toes, feet, and ankles to exhibit fluidity and hinge fully, the healthier we can become?

I've also realized how few of us want to allow our toes and the bottoms of our feet to *slowly lower* our weight into the ground as we walk. I've long been a fan of big toe pushups; I've only recently realized how lowering my weight slowly through my toes back onto the ground truly stretches and tones the under surface of my feet and massages my adrenal system. Just as the lowering motion of a pushup is work, so is allowing the return phase of a healthy toe pushup. Very few people seem to know how to push their weight off from their toes each time they step forward, or *slowly* allow its return to the earth through its toe hinge. The back leg pushes and propels the walk; then the front leg slowly lowers to contact the earth. Yet too many of us shuffle through life. This shuffle seems to suggest the attitude: "What's the use?" Others race through, barely touching the ground, in an "I'll never do enough" mode.

## I CAN DO ANYTHING

I work to instill, instead, the attitude: "I can do anything I need to do. I can and will do what it takes to succeed, achieve, and enjoy life to the fullest." Imagine walking with a "What's the use?" or an "I'll never do enough" attitude. Then imagine a walk with a relaxed "I can do anything" attitude. Which walk feels more fun? Can you feel your body shift? Can you begin to stand on your own two feet? Can you challenge those who are ready to make changes?

I've previously mentioned mentor Louis Schultz's challenge to us to go home and play with our bodies. I never heard him ask anyone to go home and work on anything. I think he was on a good track. As soon as we work on change, we've put ourselves into a win/lose situation, yet if we play with making changes, we won't fail. So *play* with standing in your toes and teach your clients to do the same. Play with walking less heavily in your heels and more joyfully springing through your toes with each step. Play with allowing the weight to shift through the various points on the bottom of your foot and let the entire foot touch the floor. And play with toning the deep muscles on the foot's lower surface with toe lifts, up *and* down. Play with massaging toes, calves, even knees and hips.

I realized again just the other day: The length of the walk I take to exercise my body is less important than the presence I bring to my walk and the ability I find to tune into my body. If I focus on using my big toe hinge more fully, allowing the little toes to follow, my entire body is engaged. When I feel my feet and enjoy my interaction with a safe and supportive earth, I can walk for five minutes, take my time, find the joy in my step, and feel relaxed. Yet I can walk for two miles or a half hour, effort to achieve a workout, and never pay attention to the way my body feels. I'm not accomplishing anything positive if I'm not living in my body when I take it for a walk.

I've also begun to massage the backs of my legs while flexing and extending my toes and ankles, and I'm teaching clients to do this for themselves. I feel I'm helping old blood and stuck energy in the feet and ankles move up through the body by gently "milking" the tibialis posterior and other calf muscles to push blood toward the heart *while* allowing the toes to move up and down. Move stuck energy! In my class, "Top Ten Hot Spots to Affect Greater Change," spot number two is tibialis posterior release (number one is psoas/diaphragm; see Chapter 3).

You can also give, or teach clients to give themselves, a reflexology treatment. If each body part has a corresponding point on the sole of the foot, stimulating the foot points will also stimulate, challenge, and release the points above (Figure 5.5). The Chinese have been using such a system for thousands of years, while we in the West have only been using it for the past hundred. I believe many of us have sore reflex points precisely where we've tried to protect our feet from touching the ground or have totally surrendered into it. Why not simply sit with foot in hand to poke, squeeze, and twist the sole to stimulate the parts above? When you or clients find a tighter or sore spot, work to rub and release it, with breath. Points most people really need to release: shoulders, spine, occiput inside the big toe, and stomach/costal arch reflex that happens to hold several TCM lines.

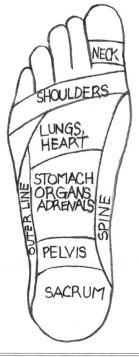

Figure 5.5 Reflexology chart
*Stimulating, but holding, points and achieving
breath creates more potent release above.*

Before you begin the next chapter, think to yourself: How secure and excited do I feel to be on this planet, in this body, at this time? Am I grounded? Am I enthusiastic and joyful to be here? Am I fearful in my world? Do I feel defeated in my life? Do I defeat myself? Answer honestly; then *play* with making changes. Only then are you ready to ask for change from your clients.

## Remember

- Most of us are physically dying from the feet up into the rest of our body. By slowing energy at the feet, we deprive everything above. Our relationship to the earth is important, yet we don't consider it as part of our health regimen.

- Many of us still try to please or imitate (but rarely do so) elders with self-limiting behaviors. We need to choose whether these behaviors truly serve, or are just habits. Either we surrender to life, fight against it, or joyfully walk through it; we're on our toes, "de-feeted," or "watching our step."

- The tibialis posterior and flexor muscles behind the two leg bones and extensor muscles just in front of them are keys to creating health, resilience, and safety in the legs and the body. Play with finding and using these deep muscles.

## All purpose cue

"Experiment with walking and standing slightly more in your toes. Allow them to hinge and push you off when standing, and especially when walking. Occasionally revert to standing and walking heavily in your heels. Can you feel the difference? Which do you prefer? Continue the experiment. Believe you could walk through life on feet that safely and happily take you wherever you want to go. Walk as though you're not in a hurry, but you're happy to be going where you're going."

## Client challenge

### EASY

Simply observe where in your feet your weight reaches the ground. Are they mirror images? Ask them to become more alike. Create flexibility and symmetry in your feet and energy in your legs. When you have a moment, observe and make a change. *Play with it.*

### MEDIUM

Can you bend the knees slightly *and* lift into a big toe pushup at the same time?

## DIFFICULT

Stand on one leg; take the other foot in your hand and pull its toes skyupbehind your body (you may need to hold a chair or table for balance). Now focus on staying balanced in the foot that contacts the earth. Once you feel reasonably solid, experiment with moving your body's weight forward and inside (bigtoeward) and feel where else this stretch tugs at your deep line—and your balance.

## INTRIGUING

Whenever you feel threatened, check to see if you're pulling your energy up and away from the ground as you "tiptoe through life." Is it more one side than the other? Can you relax and breathe?

## IMAGINE

Can you learn to begin the day with an attitude and a first step that says "I can do anything"? Can you transfer that attitude to your walk and banish fear and weariness from your step?

# THE BACK UP PLAN

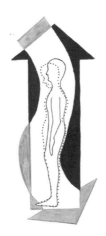

## WHO RULES—SURVIVE, OR THRIVE?

*That which we perceive as negativity causes us to*
*shorten and tighten, especially at our heads.*

In Chapter 1 I suggested we'll follow Ida Rolf and hold the top of the head up and the back of the waist back. This can happen as you go down the street, stand at the kitchen sink, or talk to a friend. In these next two chapters we'll work to put the head on straight and keep the gut from being the catch basin of unresolved feelings. While staying grounded in healthy feet, we'll find our head and waist. Other body hinges, chakras, and postures will join the equation in later chapters as we journey through the body and challenge specific segments and the emotions stored in them.

Let's visit more commonsense body wisdom: In addition to having a "good head on their shoulders," some people always want to be "head and shoulders" above everyone else. Some are praised for "having their heads on straight" or "using their head." In *my* head, we get "headed in the wrong direction" for one of several reasons: We're working hard to achieve (get ahead), we're still protecting ourselves from blows that could rain down on us (watch your head), we've clouded our brains with useless information so we can't retrieve the vital stuff (crammed our heads), or we've allowed negativity to overtake us (lost our heads).

This chapter's logo conveys my belief that we change our world by simply backing up and standing straight—getting our heads on straight to get a good look at what comes at us and reacting calmly to it, instead of shortening our essence to protect ourselves, take up less space, and "head off" the challenge.

An important trait of this chapter's up arrow symbol is its flexibility. Turn this arrow into a spine…now imagine you're looking at yourself sitting or standing sideways. Can you see the chakras jamming closer together as the head and neck pitch forward? (See Figure 6.1.) Perhaps your clients sit at a computer much of the time. Perhaps they spend lots of time in car or airplane seats, or a recliner chair. Perhaps they're just weary and feel like their head wants to fall forward off their body. How do we keep a good head on our shoulders? While we need spinal curves for shock absorbency, too many of us have overdeveloped curves; our up arrow is squashed and shortened.

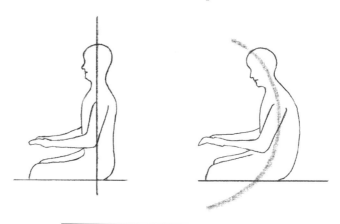

Figure 6.1 Good and bad sitting posture

*A bad sitting posture can contribute to a forward head when we stand. This in turn puts undue stress on the erector and rhomboid muscles.*

I suggest that depending on which chakra calls the shots, arrives first, or takes up space, *we* become different people in different bodies. The chakras draw energy from the ground up, from surviving to thriving: Survival (root chakra) is clearly any organism's first order of business, and reproduction or propagation (second or sacral) comes right after if we're to continue our line. The gut and heart deal with nutrition and circulation of fuel—more basic survival instincts. The throat gives voice to needs and ingests fuel. The head chakras manage and oversee proceedings. All together, if humming properly and moving from center to center easily, the lower six centers form the body; the seventh oversees the body and draws energy from the universe above; and an eighth *aura* suffuses the entire being with natural energy and allows it to thrive. Physical and emotional problems come when we get congested in any one or more of these chakras and deprive them of rightful energy—when our head and our gut get too close together.

This chapter encourages us all to operate consciously from a higher level instead of baser, lower centers. As most of us live and move from lower (guts or groin) *or* head (but usually third eye, not crown), we can become trapped in a personality directed by the most—or least—active chakra. Many of us seem afraid to allow the crown, or seventh, higher power chakra, to guide the body. The crown should be in charge of our bodymindcore: Imagine operating your body from that place situated just above your head.

For now let's focus on the sixth chakra. The brain and cranial nerves are served or starved at the third eye, located behind the eyebrows and encompassing the brain and skull, the *atlas* bone just below the occiput at the top of the spine, and the *pituitary* or master gland which controls the entire glandular system. The third eye deals with a person's ability to self-determine and make their way. It's the center of consciousness, and the place from where we're able to operate the body. My descriptive third eye phrase is "Rationally think without worry." Worry is the constant misuse of energy for fearful reasons. We worry when we become greedy: Will there be enough for me? Can I be charitable? We often make our decisions from this worry chakra without regard to the larger perspective our higher seventh chakra thinking brings. When one gets too tied up in the third eye one may become ungrounded and unfocused or too cerebral—the brain may feel fuzzy or, conversely, that it has to manage every detail of the universe.

Think back to the three main Oriental dantian centers: the head, heart, and stomach. We've also mentioned three burners, at the heart, stomach, and pelvic bowl. The complicated old Chinese system features four centers instead of seven chakras; heart and gut are basic to both, and we run energy through our diaphragm hourglass by lifting our head and dropping our tail back and out of it, thus stretching our elastic band in several directions.

A tight, tired, overworked, or closed sixth chakra may create overwhelming negativity or a "What's the use?" attitude. Problems arising from tension or shortness of the head and neck might include, but certainly aren't limited to: headaches, strokes, lack of concentration up to dementia, attention deficit/hyperactivity disorder, extreme sensitivity, and impairment of vision, hearing, taste, smell, and balance. On the positive side, when we stretch this area, we're able to create more of a "Yes, I can" attitude in our bodymindcore that enhances the feet's "I can do anything" attitude.

## WHY AM I IN PAIN?

Recently I began working with Judy, another new client who lives in pain. I often ask such a client to quantify their pain level on a scale of one to ten: one is easily tolerable and ten is "I can't stand to live in this body." Judy responded that she lives in a ten daily. I've lived with intense pain, and to me, at number three or four I begin to have a "fuzzy" head; 30–40 percent of my energy is used to cope, and little reaches my head. Six is the marker where I have trouble functioning physically, and eight is the place I might consider suicide. If I were living at a ten, with 100 percent of my energy devoted to my pain, I doubt I'd be able to get out of bed, much less get myself to an appointment.

Without invalidating her experience, I wonder: What in one's emotional makeup causes such physical pain? Is this a *psychosomatic* (all in her head) pain, or a *somatopsychic* (vivid trauma that makes her mentally unstable) pain? In addition to physical pain, Judy's personal life has fallen apart; yet she has a firm belief that it's her purpose to stay on the planet. Can I help her improve her life? I think so.

Pain is resistance to change. I believe we spend too much time hiding or protecting ourselves from or resisting change. The pain we know is ours, and we've learned how to tolerate it and carry on. What's on the other side of that pain? We're afraid to go through it and find out, so resist investigating. We've got to learn to go below the current pain into that which hurt us deeply and early. We've got to find it, feel it, look it in the eye, and soften and release it. Chronic pain seems to illustrate the axiom that we can't go around emotional injuries; to heal we must go through them.

Our pain desensitizes us emotionally and physically. Our brain recognizes pain and tries to mask it, yet focuses on what we don't want. We resist delving further into ourselves to examine, acknowledge, lick our wounds, strengthen and heal, then re-enter society. Instead, we shorten and pull into ourselves.

Our lower six chakras tighten everywhere and build a full-scale concrete bunker around and about the traumas we've experienced. If we refuse to look at and acknowledge the bad things we've seen and endured, we hope we'll control them and they'll lose their power over us. We cover over the emotional charge around our old issues, and focus on a thought form: "PAIN! Stay away." Psychologists would probably call this state "denial," or describe the individual as "very defended."

Recently I've been focusing on two phrases. The first challenges us to look at "our weary fears." I think most of us live in fear of what *has* happened or *might* happen to us, based on our past. Our fears are weary because we've held them for so long…in some cases, we're no longer even aware we have them; yet they still control us. We must acknowledge weary fears if we want to move through to freedom. My second new phrase is "Your pain has lost its voice." A student told me she'd recently suffered a tailbone injury and gone for medical treatment. Her doctor warned her that the injury would hurt a long time. What will heal it? I think without intervention and acknowledgment, nothing will heal it; she'll just eventually stop noticing it. When her pain has screamed so long and so hard that it realizes no one is listening, it will become a deep, silent whimper—a weary fear and voiceless stuck energy, resisting change.

## EXPLORING OUR PAIN

My best sessions with clients come about when I get them to work with me; identifying, stretching, and bringing breath into their painful places. We create a partnership that encourages them to learn to acknowledge and release their pain themselves, instead of waiting for someone to do it for or to them.

Judy and I have begun exploring her coping process by asking her to stay present while I show her *where* her pain lives in her body. As I touch painful places, I ask her to stretch her breath and her tissues through her pain and fear. She's been amazed to realize that if she acknowledges her pain's voice, often pain finally releases its grip on her. Like Judy, too many of us deny our pain's message, so we hurt even more.

When I see a new client, nearly 100 percent of the time the first place I want to touch is Chapter 3's area of the chest just below the heart at the diaphragm muscle. Here I can usually make the biggest change in a client's ability to have a deep, cleansing breath. If I can help them open their heart/gut "hourglass" gateway, I've already helped them begin to lengthen their head, neck, and shoulders by stretching the shortened connective tissue that travels up the front of the spine and the back of the breastbone. If we simply learn to lengthen the back of our necks by straightening and lifting our heads, many dis-eases might not find a place to live. I often tell clients moss won't grow where the sun shines and the wind blows.

Unresolved traumas and feelings may cause the spine to lose its pliability and leave "kinks" and sharper curves somewhere in its up arrow. Relaxed lifting headlong allows energy and circulation to reach all the way to the head. The long muscles up the back—the *erector spinae* (of the spine)—help to hold the head high (Figure 6.2). Deep to erectors, short muscles tie individual spinal segments together. Curves in our spine are good, but short and tight curves that steal the overall length of the spine are harmful. We begin opening these curves by lifting our head as we breathe.

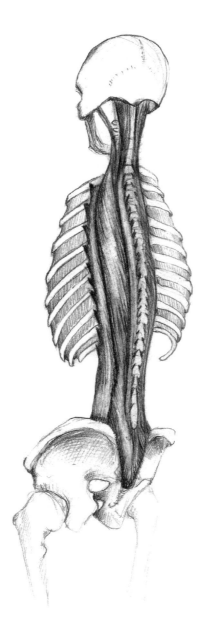

Figure 6.2 Erector spine

*The erector spinae group could create span and length instead
of tension and shortness. Remove some of the spinal curves
by standing with the head up and the waist back.*

As I said earlier, I believe we die physically from the feet up; I think we die *mentally* from the head down. As we tighten our head and neck, energy can't nurture them. The hourglass I earlier described between gut and heart is mirrored by a secondary one between head and neck…when the "sand" here gets stuck and the spine gets pulled short and tight, our heads get clouded. Without energy to the head, we're less able to think, to do, or be.

Headaches of any sort (particularly migraines) often come about because, due to physical or mental tension, the blood vessels to the head have constricted and aren't allowing circulation between the head and body. With tension in the head and neck it's difficult for blood to retreat back through this upper hourglass toward the body. If we could just move that static blood in the head, much of what we call migraines, and possibly even strokes, might be averted.

As you observe people around you, chances are you'll notice many who live with their heads out front. I often contrast the general and the foot soldier for clients—the general sits at the top of the hill and feels safely supported at all times as he directs the action below…the foot soldier sticks his neck out and gets his head blown off. Which head do you wear? How does it feel?

## UNRESOLVED THOUGHT FORMS

When someone drinks or uses drugs, or has a very negative personality, it's often said the person "has a demon." This may be truer than we'd considered. Perhaps there *are* energetic demons clinging to us. What if some of our behaviors are from external energy that's become attached to us? What if these behaviors or thoughts push our heads downfront and stop us from "lifting our eyes to the hills, from whence comes our help" (Psalm 121:1)?

What some might call demons or entities, I've long called "negative thought forms." I've begun to reframe them as unresolved, disturbed, or *unprocessed* thought forms. This helps me accept responsibility for whatever has come into my world. A thought's energy may have been pitched to me by someone else: positive or negative, disembodied or not; I caught it and didn't let it go. Whether it's mine or someone else's, I need to learn how to consciously choose whether to allow its energy to remain in my life and body.

And please understand: Whatever name we give to the energies of thought forms, they are real. Energy is real, and stuck energy is a real problem. Whether positive or negative energy is sent to us by others, it's our challenge to process and release it from our bodymindcores. We can't see gravity, yet we accept that it's real. Energy is just as real as gravity; some of us are only beginning to understand this law.

I believe among the worst places to pick up unresolved thought forms are bars, hospitals, and other places of mental confusion and anxiety where people in turmoil are more susceptible to fear, negativity, or mental abandon. Finding such a weakened state, this unresolved thought energy can easily attach itself. Any negative place or situation can cause such traumas. Can we learn to release these negative energies which come at us and threaten to overwhelm us?

## ATLAS WEDGE

When unresolved thought energies attach, they often create an *atlas wedge* at the back of the neck and just under the head. This attachment shortens the neck so the *atlas* bone (the first cervical bone or C1) jams forward, kinking the spine, choking the spinal column, causing an energetic slowdown to the head and a lack of nerve conduction to the body, and squeezing the occipital bone toward the *axis* or second cervical bone as the head pitches forward (Figure 6.3). The brain loses some communication and becomes unsure of the body, so the lower chakras retreat into survival mode. If we can lift our head upback out of these energetic thought forms and breathe to release, we can "get our heads on straight" and clean our channel again.

An atlas wedge shortens and chokes the *animal* brain—the oldest part of our brain, the stem in the neck which, like lower chakras, deals with survival and security. When this animal brain is under constant pressure, how can we possibly live a full and happy life? Yet when we stretch and straighten our head—lifting it *and* settling it back and on top of our body—we create space and circulation in the survival brain and allow energy to the *pituitary* gland. Since this gland both manages the entire glandular system and the growth and aging process, doesn't it make sense to lift our head instead of pulling into ourselves, shortening and trapping our energy and causing us to spin our wheels and age faster?

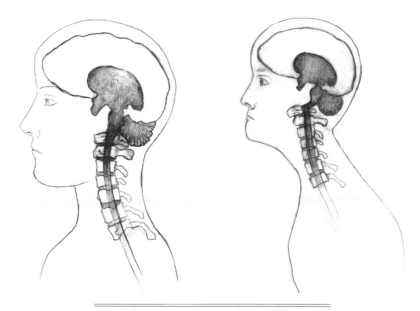

Figure 6.3 Good (L) and bad (R) atlas wedge

*A bad atlas wedge occurs when the first cervical bone (atlas) gets pinched forward and the spinal column is choked, depriving the head and brain of energy.*

It's a good concept: That which we perceive as negativity causes us to shorten and tighten our heads (as well as our hearts, our guts, and our groins). We shorten the front line of our body (emotions) and our head rides around in front of us, causing our physical back pain. By releasing negative energies, or not allowing them in the first place, we keep our head on straight. By emulating the straight arrow symbol we invite opening, lengthening, and cleaning of our neck and spine tension, release of negative thought forms, and energy to the head. By modeling it, we encourage it in our clients.

## CORE fascial release of head/back of neck: Head on straight

1. Client supine, cradle head with one or two hands, preferably one at occiput and one on chin.

2. Monitor the client's breath. First, find some. When you feel their breath rhythm, challenge it slightly. Each time client exhales, give a mild traction.

3. Feel for client's breath challenging the restriction you've created. If you can't feel that breath breakthrough, lighten your traction slightly and try again.

4. When you feel, or even intuit, client breath coming through, add a bit of traction. Coax client, for two to three minutes, to breathe and release this unresolved tension.

5. This is a good way to end any and every session.

6. Remember, you can choose to remain free of whatever unresolved stuff your client releases!

If we don't release these thought forms we'll be depressed, or find an addiction that numbs us so we don't feel the pain of living with them. But if we acknowledge we have unresolved thought forms (pain/resistance to change) stuck in us, we can begin the process of dissolving that which shortens us into ourselves. Let's work to remove unresolved trauma—old and new—as soon as possible.

## MAKING HEADWAY

Identify and release negative energies which may have adhered to you; stretch your neck, then teach clients to find and stretch their own: "Lengthen the back of your neck by arching your head upback long-overforward *while* neck stays rounded back; then draw half circles or crescents with your head, allowing your shoulders and spine to follow. When you find a spot that tugs or hurts, gently and respectfully see if you can create a bit more stretch, breath, and movement in that area."

Here's a client awareness to help reverse all the head forward activities we practice far too much of the time: "Stand about one foot out from a wall, with your back to it. Lean your shoulders into the wall; allow your head to touch it also. Lift/pull/stretch your shoulders away from the wall in various directions while staying connected to the floor with your feet and to the wall with the back of your head. Can you feel how this line opens the shoulders as it restores your head to its rightful position on top of your body?" (See Figure 6.4.)

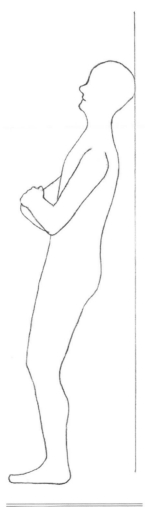

Figure 6.4 Head on a wall

*A simple (not easy!) stretch to reduce head and back pressures.*

Help your clients get their heads on straight. It really is as simple (not easy!) as reminding self, "top of the head up." The more we can "upback" our neck and "uplong" our head, the less pain and negativity can get stuck in a tense head or spine, and the more energy can flow through our entire being and allow us to keep a good head on our shoulders. In any succeeding chapter or exercise, in your practice, or at any time, lift *your* head above the rest of the body.

## Remember

- Think of pain as resistance to change and an unresolved thought form. When we're stuck, it's often because we're afraid to go forward, into, and through our pain.

- If we visualize a straight up arrow in our spine, we realize most of us have a "kink" or curve near the top of the spine: our head and neck don't fit happily on top, or are too rigid. Simply bringing our head and neck upback begins to change the way we operate and *feel* in the world.

- Storing unresolved energetic and emotional thought forms is a subtle way we screw our heads down too tightly. We can choose whether to store these negative thoughts that pull us down, or to let them move through and out of us.

## All purpose cue

"Check into your own physical, energetic, and emotional state. Then place your hands behind your head and tug your chin toward your chest and your forehead toward your knees *while* you push the back of your neck into a curve away from you. You can do the same thing lying on the ground—just bring your head forward and your neck back. After you breathe and stretch, check your own energetic levels again."

# Client challenge

### Simple

Whenever you think of it, lift your head up and your waist back.

### Medium

Let's take the spinal arrow and put length in it: Lie on your back, on the floor. Let your heels and inner arches reach as long and far away from your body as you can get them. Now, pull your neck and head long *while* your back stays floorback. Breathe!

### Difficult

Now change positions; roll onto your stomach and raise yourself on your elbows (you'll be happier on a pad or mattress than on a harder surface). Let your head move uplong (twisting if you want) *while* the belly button and groin pull earthdownlong, *while* you open your heart, *while* you shift weight from elbow to elbow. Pull your head out of your heart; then out of your low back; finally out of your tail.

### Intriguing

Who or what have you allowed to "get in *your* head" and attach negatively to you? Can you make a change?

### Imagine

As you become familiar with the chakra model, which chakra(s) do you think hold their breath in *your* body? Which governs, and which hides?

# CHAPTER 7

# TRUST YOUR GUT

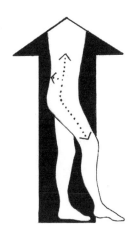

## THE CHURN—JUDGE, OR DISCERN?

*Why not learn to dis-charge our stuck energy traumas more
immediately instead of nursing them along through the years?*

How did we get knots in our stomach, and how do we untie them?
Jonathan relived a tailbone injury as we worked to release old patterns
in his body. He remembered being a young child in the country and
"bouncing" down a flight of concrete stairs on his tailbone. The pain
from this trauma didn't strike me as unusual. His mother's response
seemed strange, however.

She immediately picked Jonathan up by the heels and shook him
until she got him gulping and gasping for breath. Isn't it a great
picture of a little boy being held upside down by the ankles and being
shaken until he screamed? Her intention was probably to shake breath
and spinal realignment into him; I suspect she shook the breath *out*
of him instead. While her intention was to help and heal him, did she

help or hinder? We often hurt the ones we love: At least she didn't do it in anger, as too many do.

When I first heard this story I thought, "How primitive." Yet Mama had a clear goal to immediately confront a block in her son's physical and emotional body—an unresolved thought energy—and shake that block loose before it had time to settle. I wish she'd have said, with a mother's love: "You'll be fine...shake it out, relax, and breathe." Too many well-meaning parents try to teach their children to disown and disavow the reality of trauma experiences. They ask their child to store or stifle trauma instead of finding a way to help them loosen and release.

We're taught to immediately try to neutralize incoming messages instead of examining them fearlessly. Our attempts to strengthen our children with stern words often only pitch more disturbed thought forms at them, shortening their heads and storing trauma deeper inside them—anchoring fear in a tight gut.

"You're not hurt—pick yourself up."

"You stop crying or I'll give you something to cry about."

"Don't be a sissy."

"Nobody likes a crybaby."

"You're not dead!"

Too many of us spend our lives treating children, spouses/partners, and sometimes even parents in ways that discourage the release of trauma and encourage the storing of it in the gut. If we can't learn to sort through this emotional dump of past traumas, we'll eventually be buried in its garbage. How can we teach our children their blocks are self-perpetuated, even when they're other-imposed?

I'm reminded how many of us either "spill our guts" or "tie our stomach in knots." We "can't stomach" some people or "get sick to our stomach" at the prospect of certain situations. Some of us fill our guts to obesity, or starve ourselves; possibly as a protection against external influences we can't control any other way. In traditional chakra models the adrenal glands are connected to this gut. As this gland has the ability to allow us to decide if a threat is real or imagined, it's gut-level important. When an animal senses danger, its adrenal system instructs it either to run from the danger, stand and fight, go numb, or decide all is safe and shake out those danger signals.

Why can't we do that?

Learning to allow the waist to stay back and level while the upper back stays upback develops awareness in the solar plexus: the stomach, colon, liver, kidneys, spleen, and digestive system. Problems which may arise here include IBS (irritable bowel syndrome), irregularity of the bowel, diabetes, kidney failure, weight management problems, eating disorders, glandular irregularity, and many low back issues. The gland I'd associate with this chakra is the pancreas; though many would argue it's an organ, its function might be seen as the regulation of sweetness through one's life—the production and release of insulin is very much a chemical and glandular function, and our overuse of sugar may just have something to do with our need for sweetness in our lives. The most important organs in this center, and indeed, some would say the body, are the kidneys. If we don't process and eliminate the unresolved through the gut, energy slows and we become ill.

I think we've lost integrity and discernment in this stomach chakra. How can we get better at finding and honoring our guts, and teaching our children to do the same? Consider: When this particular energy center gets clogged and the back tightens, the gut arrives to meet the world first. Too true for too many of us—we're shortening our backs and our lives.

Do *you* relax your guts and enjoy integrity, personal power, and self-esteem? Can you be comfortable in your gut, being who you are? Or do you continually try to be, or pretend to be, someone else? Can you be patient, or are you angry? The chakra phrase I employ to describe this third center is "Honestly discern without judgment." Judgment is the acceptance of your fear that you aren't good enough, and the need to prove to others, at their expense, that you are. Too many of us judge because we've been taught to do so. If we stop judging self, we let go of our judgments of clients and create space for them to heal.

## JUDGMENT AND DISCERNMENT

Without judging my or another's behavior as wrong, it's still possible for me to discern whether a behavior enhances my life or another's, then whether I want to maintain that particular behavior. I don't need to make someone wrong to decide where they are or where they're going isn't where I want to be. It's not my job to change their behavior, unless I see it harming someone who doesn't yet have the skills to say "no" to an older or stronger individual. It's not my job to free someone else from old patterns unless they ask for help. It's my job to discern whether someone else's behavior, or mine, lengthens or shortens my bodymindcore, and to challenge clients to do likewise.

Discernment is honest surrender to and appraisal of the movement of *authentic energy* through the bodymindcore. Does a thought lengthen and relax tissues (yes, good, you're on the right path); or shorten and tighten them (no, go another way)? We can feel the difference. Discernment can tell us much, if we'll listen. Decide to keep track of how often you overrule your discernment. Begin asking for truer discernment—gut to crown—as you learn to stay out of judgment mode. Learn to truly discern what's enhancing your life and what's stifling your vital capacity. When you release judgment in favor of discernment you're already a greater aid to your clients.

Each of us needs to let go of self-judgment *and* judgment by others (censorship), and instead rely on self-discernment, which listens to the gut but allows the crown to rule. We need to discern who we are, what we need, and what's good or bad, wrong or right for us, independent of what society tells us we need to become. We can claim—and express—our core authority.

## HURTING THE ONES WE LOVE

All of us grew up with interesting personal family patterns—many based on fear and competition. We learned to hurt each other. Why? Why do we hurt those we love, and why do those we love hurt us? We learned such destructive behaviors from damaged elders who accepted the teaching you can't expect too much joy in your life, and you might as well get that truth trained into you early. You'll probably never have enough, do enough, or be good enough. Many families pass this consciousness through generations and unconsciously live this core-tightening belief. Scarcity and powerlessness consciousness have no place in child rearing, partnering, or anything that's supposed to look like love. Our negative beliefs get stuck in our children's guts as well as our own.

We all compete for positive regard. Ridicule, criticism, and shaming are competitive tools we've learned from elders who tried to shape us. We learn to disbelieve we could or should approve of self as much as we do others.

If such competitive spirit weren't in the world there'd be tolerance and respect. I push you to join me so I can say, "See? I'm right! Look at those who agree!" If I feel secure in my religion, I'm free to let you practice yours. If I feel secure in my sexuality, I have less interest in how you express yours. If I feel secure in my family, I stop competing for attention and enjoy what comes to me. This competitive spirit is difficult to change, since it's consistently reinforced. But when we stop competing for love or external positive regard, believe we deserve it, and so give it to ourselves first, the world changes. We see each situation as an opportunity instead of a threat.

Someone who locks in a judgment at gut level that his fundamental beliefs and behaviors are correct, valid, and necessary isn't usually interested in being challenged or informed by others. While the gut may still discern doubt, he's put a protective shell over core labeled "no change." He may discern his "gut feeling" is wrong, but he honors what he judges and chooses to believe what the gut tells him. Judgment ties our stomach in knots; discernment allows us to stay open.

## ENCOURAGING DISCHARGE

Years ago I attended a reflective listening seminar that helped untrained people band together in partnerships to uncover and discharge old mental and emotional traumas. I found it changed my parenting and my bodywork. For a specified time period, one partner is client and the other is listener. As the client discharges, the listener restates what they hear: "So, you're feeling sad about that?" There's no judgment of feelings offered, only self-discernment encouraged.

Reflective listening allows the "client" to process their issues at their chosen level and speed, to dislodge and discharge any stuck trauma or unresolved thought form that's slowing their energy. At the end of a specified time period, roles are switched and the listener becomes client. It can be effective, affordable therapy with one rule: No advice! Empathetic restatement of the client's thoughts to coax further discharge is the only acceptable feedback.

When I found this technique I already knew my past was shaping my present, and that, unexamined, it would continue to shape my future, not necessarily in a direction I wanted to go. In addition to making me diligent in my quest to know what had caused sadness and fear in my early years, examining my old traumas also got me questioning *my* parenting skills with our two-year-old. Why not encourage her to discharge small unpleasant traumas more immediately instead of nursing them along through the years? Why not help the two-year-old face the trauma, feel the feelings, and work through and release them to go forward with clean energy?

Immediate discharge helps. I remember specific instances of holding my young daughter and saying, "Wow, you're really sad (or hurt, or angry) right now, aren't you? You just need to cry a bit, don't you? Well, let me hold on while you get that out. Go ahead, let it out!" I don't remember saying, "Stop crying! You're a big girl now and it wasn't that bad!" I encouraged movement of unhappy feelings, to discharge more immediately instead of holding her trauma. I remember times when she cried horribly for ten minutes, then sniffled, cleared her eyes and lungs, and happily went off to play, problem forgotten! I invite all parents to consider this model... I only wish mine had heard of it, and I wish I'd remembered it through her teen years.

In the present, I occasionally examine and release old fears with the memory of my long-departed grandfather. As I remember him, I ask him to advocate for me in uncomfortable situations, as together we soothe my damaged and unsettled pieces. Did someone in your family of origin pour healing waters on your tears when you were a kid? Could they advocate for you now? Do you trust anyone from unhappy times to stand with you? Feel their strength and resolve in *your* gut.

No matter what experience is coming, I hope to trust my gut and allow the experience to come into and *move through me as quickly as possible.* I believe with all my heart: The more quickly and fearlessly we're able to acknowledge any stimulus or thought energy, no matter how harsh, in an open and receptive mood, the quicker we process and release it from our consciousness so it's not stuck in our bodymindcore. And if it won't move, we're emotionally and energetically constipated.

If we can teach our children how to trust their discernment to acknowledge trauma, then dissolve and work through it at their gut, we've done great parenting. If we can further coax them to allow *every* energy to move through them with discernment and without judgment, they'll have fewer knots in their stomachs. And if we can practice discernment in our life and model it for theirs, it'll have a positive and healing effect on our clients as well as our children.

## PSOAS—PRIMARY STORER OF ALL STRESS

One muscle covers a great deal of the front of the lower and middle spine on each of us; it proceeds in front of our pubic bone and dives down into the deep inside and middle of our leg, where it anchors at the lesser trochanter. Its primary purpose is to maintain the front of our body, but it tightens our back and allows us to stay short at the gut. It's the muscle I believe ties our stomach in knots *and* gives us backaches. Since the muscle covers so much ground, it also shows us why this third chakra area is vital to overall health and well-being. Remember, the classical Oriental medicine model sees the back of the back as more symptomatic of physical manifestations and the front relates to emotional ones. Whether Chinese, Indian, or Western, many of us recognize the importance of the front of the back. Yet many massage schools discourage touching the area.

I'm intrigued with *psoas*, and I've created an acronym for it— PSOAS: Primary Storer Of All Stress. I believe every hit we've ever taken—physical, mental, emotional, chemical, electrical, energetic— are all stuck and stored in that psoas muscle behind the gut (Figure 7.1); unless and until someone is wise enough to convince us to let these traumas go, or unless someone who parented us was already wise enough to encourage more immediate trauma release.

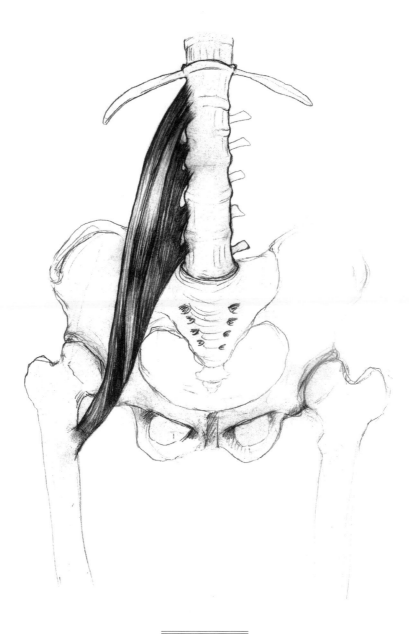

Figure 7.1 Psoas

*From the lesser trochanter of the thigh all the way to T12, the psoas is the lightning rod that shortens our entire being when it's under stress. Consider its connection to the diaphragm: Health resides in creating a relaxed relationship between them.*

A healthy psoas is toned but not too tight, and knows how to lengthen, loosen, and fall back with every step. Many of us have extremely tight psoas muscles, from working hard to hold it together, keep it in, tiptoe through life, or shorten our back to stand our ground (Figure 7.2). A healthy psoas relaxes when we stand or walk. An overtightened psoas pulls our low back forward, spills guts downout, and even pitches the head and neck forward off our body (head upback!). As we relax *and* retone psoas muscles, we create a new healthier posture and mental attitude.

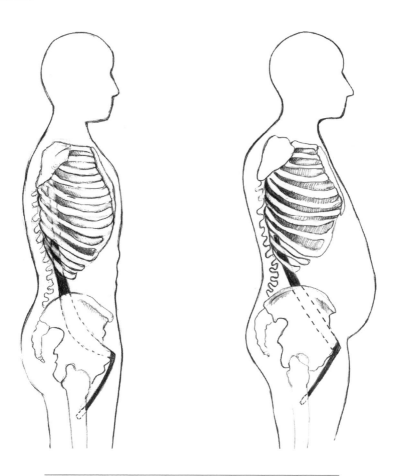

Figure 7.2 Healthy (L) and unhealthy (R) psoas muscles

*Note how a tight and/or weak psoas can pull the low back anterior, allow the rectus to lose tone, and cause the head to pull forward.*

This chapter's logo shows an upback arrow at the waist, on an upward spine/arrow, *while* a leg lengthens. I'm convinced the more we learn to live with our waist tucked upback *while* we move, the more we'll exercise our psoas with every step and every breath. As we maintain a better posture through life, the longer and healthier our life can be.

## CORE fascial release of lower psoas

1.  Client supine, legs down flat, if they can do so comfortably.

2.  One sided: Palpate near belly button (L1/2), outside of rectus. Allow fingers to sink in toward spine at 45 degree angle, until you feel the client's body restrict you.

3.  Call for small movement with breath; same, then other side leg draws *incrementally* up and down, one at a time.

4.  Second touch inside hipbone at about ASIS (anterior superior iliac spine), then outside rectus and toward low spine, about L4/5.

5.  Call for same and other side legs again; you may find a different pattern.

6.  Side two with same protocol.

7.  Chances are one psoas and the opposite iliacus are tight.

We already worked to release the upper psoas as it gets tied to the lower diaphragm cords at T12/L2 in Chapter 3. As you learn to release the lower psoas, you're definitely changing a client's discernment.

Give this simple awareness to clients: "Lie on the floor or bed, on your back. Pull your own low back downback—imagine you can suck your belly button down into your back. Now, keeping your back floorback and keeping your head and neck outlongback, gently drag one heel toward your body so your knee reaches toward the ceiling *while* it also reaches uplong away from your hip." (It's important for you to experience this feeling so you can teach it to clients.) "You may or may not feel a deep line stretch; even so you're toning that deep psoas muscle. Can you do the same exercise while telling yourself you're all right, just as you are? Can you release unresolved thought energy?" (See Figure 7.3.)

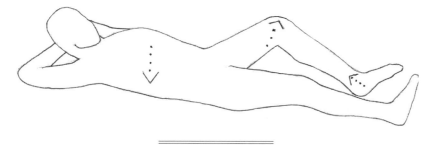

Figure 7.3 Psoas drag

*An all purpose stretch that could help any low back.*
*Remember to keep the navel into the floor/table when*
*dragging the heel and bringing the knee ceiling ward.*

Pierre Pallardy, in his book *Gut Instinct* (2006), suggests that nearly every condition one can imagine probably begins with problems in the gut. He has an interesting chart of areas of the stomach to massage for particular maladies as well as exercises to resolve specific conditions. It's a thought-provoking book.

Imagine you can stand and stretch *your* head up and your low/mid back upback at the same time, to lengthen and tone the psoas. We just considered this line in a lying down position. Does this posture make you feel ready to face the world, or does it feel uncomfortable? Leveling the waist *while* the back stays upback seems to also allow the anus to drop down, as if you had a heavy tail. I believe this lengthening/dropping stimulates the *vagus nerve*, which allows the entire body to relax, and balances the front and back meridians. Experiment with your tail pulling long past your genitals, but keep your head up, your waist back, and your tail long as you move on to other chapters.

Sometimes I'll encourage clients to practice a very few sit ups in slow motion, *while* that waist tries to stay back. While I'm normally not a fan of sit ups, I believe if we use them slowly and ask each segment of the body to waken, they serve us. It's a worthy goal to identify individual segments of tension and release/lengthen these segments.

For the client, and for us: "Stand and bend forward, with fingertips or even palms on the floor if possible. Lift your low back ceilingup, and slowly stack spinal segment on segment. Can you create a feeling of stacking each block on the one below as you realign yourself on the way up?" This simple awareness will also help clients learn to identify, lengthen, and use both the psoas and individual low back components to soften the guts while stretching the Oriental Governing Vessel (GV) on the back of the body.

I believe the emotional content of this third chakra is too often paralysis and dread which keeps us bound in judgment. The guts feel constantly judged by the brain—did I do enough? Am I good enough? Will I have enough? Yet if we can keep our waist back and stay relaxed instead of charged in the psoas, we're better able to discern life as an adventure to be enjoyed instead of judging it as a series of trials that must be endured. We remember we can and we will enjoy life.

Can we choose to impart this idea to our children?

And remember the digestive system of the body. We take in nutrition, but for too many of us, we consume "junk" food. Due to our lack of exercise and limited intake of water, this junk gets stuck inside us. We can't process and eliminate it, so it either gets trapped in our gut or goes right through without giving us any nutrition. When we're unaware, our thoughts and feelings behave the same way. Negative, "junk" thoughts can get stuck in our guts and constipate our bodymindcore.

## STEPPING OUT OF FEAR

I challenge us all to rise out of fear (chakras 1–3) and stay out of it; to lead our children, and our clients, into discerning fearlessness also. When we can more quickly call each event good, and even when we don't yet see or understand its goodness, we'll more quickly see what that good is and how we can use it to enhance our lives. Yet if we live as if every experience is designed to cause us grief, shame, and fear, we'll be right. The choice is ours—do we want to live in a shortened and fearful body with stomachs tied in knots, or do we want to process that which fuels us and eliminate the waste while remaining open at the core? Do we treat our guts with respect or as slaves to be used up and discarded? Fear constipates us.

If you're already stepping into that which you fear, go a bit more bravely. If you're afraid to face your pain, take small first steps and praise yourself for attempting them. If you're raising children, encourage them to look at their pain more quickly and fearlessly, and help them discern how to replace old hurts with joy. If you're working with clients, encourage them to see change as a positive experience. Shake it out! If our parents didn't give us this message, it's not too late to give it to ourselves, and foster it in our clients. When we decide pain indicates change is needed, our good can be revealed.

Let's repeat this simple and profound cue: As we sit, stand, or walk, we can learn to live with our waist back and head up. No matter what activity or posture we engage in, simply allowing the waist to relax back allows our guts to soften and let energy flow through.

I invite you to try living your life with this idea at the CORE; then share it with your clients: True strength resides in the gut. Learn to trust your gut feelings, yet look for good even when a stimulus feels bad, and learn to let life flow through you. Choose to feel the nutrition in each situation; take it in, use it, process it, and eliminate it. Then move on. Stop shaking your trauma in, as Jonathan's mother did, as many other parents did, and do, and learn to shake it out and get on with your life ever more joyfully.

## Remember

- Too many of us force our children to stifle or disown trauma instead of experiencing it, learning from it, and releasing it. Too many of us are still living around our old gut traumas. A stomach that's learned to tie itself into knots may contribute to digestive and eliminative problems as well as back pain and other physical *and* emotional problems.

- In conscious parenting we examine habits and behaviors from our past that either teach our children how to process and move trauma, or how to store it.

- The psoas muscle can be referred to with the acronym PSOAS: Primary Storer Of All Stress. It acts as a lightning rod that absorbs trauma, shortening the entire body as it holds this stress. This muscle ties the stomach in knots and tugs the waist and back forward.

- Learning to hold the head upback while the waist stays back and level (not forced back), thus learning what up and back look and feel like, can change the way we stand, think, feel, be, and do.

## All purpose cue

"Practice your daily routine with your back back. Simply imagine you can keep your stomach tucked in, waist level, and head up; soften your knees, stay in your toes, and breathe! When you can truly walk with your waist back so your psoas muscle relaxes and lengthens instead of tightening with each step, it's a different world. Just think, 'On task, waist back.'"

## Client challenge

### EASY

Hold onto a waist-level railing or counter. Allow yourself to sink into one heel; anchor at the railing while your waist pulls upbackaway, making half circle undulations with your back as you keep it back and pull your waist out of your heel.

### MEDIUM

Stand, and allow your body to form a backward arch. Tighten your gluteal muscles and pull your low back forwardupback, then drop your weight into the knees and big toes. Stretch the Conception Vessel (CV) as your upper body moves upback in an arch.

## DIFFICULT

Sit in an armchair. Place both hands on one arm of the chair and twist in that direction *while* keeping the other side's waist back in the chair, *while* lifting the head. Breathe. Remember to try the other side, too. Now, push your waist forward, tighten your gluteal muscles, and shorten your back as tightly as you can. Breathe!

## INTRIGUING

Pay attention to people and situations that cause your stomach to tighten. Can you decide whether you want to avoid them (flight), confront them (fight), placate them (tie yourself in knots), or process them (eliminate the feeling) and move on? Going numb is no longer an option.

## IMAGINE

Dr. Rolf is reputed to have suggested that maturity is the ability to discern finer and finer distinctions. Can you allow yourself to mature in your body?

# SHAME IS OPTIONAL

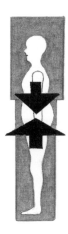

## FORBIDDEN ZONE—ASHAMED, OR AFLAME?

*What did love, or seeming positive energy directed toward you, look and feel like the first time someone shared their sexual energy with you?*

*I'm grateful for and excited by the one I've got.*

As we've planted our feet joyfully on the ground, then lifted our head and found backback, let's move to perhaps *the* most congested spot in most bodies—our genitals. Many of us believe our sexual apparatus is shameful. We seem able to talk about bowel habits more easily than we discuss sexual wants, needs, and feelings with others, whether others are lovers or strangers. Since we're embarrassed or shamed by how poorly we understand and practice sex, it's lost some of its power to serve and soothe us. I'd like us to consider how we could enjoy sexual energy, responsibly, yet free of shame.

To make up for our lack of joyful sexual energy movement, we may fantasize on the mysterious perfect sexual partner or encounter, and may or may not achieve satisfaction even there. We seem afraid to truly examine deeply what sex is about, what we do with it, or how we learn to spiritually enjoy our sexuality. Most simply, we have to learn to like ourselves unconditionally to enjoy shameless sexual feelings and/or partnerships. We've got to figure out how to celebrate our own sexual being before we share it happily with others.

I'm reminded of the early Elvis Presley. When he first appeared on the scene, grinding his pelvis to the music, much of the world was scandalized. Yet he became a sensation; perhaps exactly because he seemed able to naturally exhibit his pelvis without shame *or* pride. He was just being Elvis. I don't think he tried to be sexy, but to be Elvis. That self-security toward his sexual nature seems to have taken the world by storm. Even today, Elvis is king for many.

I've been privileged to work with some amazing clients who shared tremendous physical and emotional pain, anchored in inappropriate sexual initiation or touch that's caused them deep energetic and emotional problems for many years. It feels invasive to share too intimately these personal stories. I'll briefly create one general, representative story. It's amazing how many people (women, mostly, as I look back) refer to the pelvic or sexual area of their body as "down there." I first realized this when "Anna" said she'd never realized you could breathe or feel "down there." She represents many of us: We don't know what to make of the area "down there."

I used to observe, or believe I observed, that, like Anna, female clients were primarily bound in the pelvis, and men were bound around the heart. In my coming of age, teen girls were prone to exhibit their chests and tails; teenage boys responded with thrusting groins and closed hearts. Perhaps times have changed for some, probably not for all. These days, I perceive most of us bound up in heart *and* groin, regardless of gender. Chakra models usually suggest we must have healthy lower chakras before upper ones can open; we can't be healthy above without energy flow below. It makes sense that we need to survive before we can thrive. Before we can fully open the heart, head, or gut, we must express sexual energy creatively and be comfortable with our sexual being. We need to develop a "green line" instead of a "gray line" in our "groin line" so energy can flow through the entire being.

Sexual and reproductive problems as well as bladder and kidney issues all may occur when we aren't present "down there." We may manifest cancer, difficult periods or pregnancies, prostrate problems, lymphedema, varicosities, or endometriosis at least in part because we don't know how to allow positive energy "down there" and instead live in shame and judgment.

Often when I work with clients, I challenge them to stack their "blocks" or body parts in a new way, reaching their fingertips skyupback, then thrusting their pelvis forwarddownout, forcing themselves to recognize and feel sexual energy. This simple exercise embarrasses and stops many people. Try it…perhaps you'd rather not let energy run to the pelvis, or acknowledge it in any way. Does something bubble up to your stomach, where judgment tells sexual energy to "go away!"?

## THE ONLY DIS-EASE

I truly believe and often restate: The only dis-ease is the slowdown of energy, Paracelsus' congestion. Wilhelm Reich, psychotherapist student of Sigmund Freud and mentor to Alexander Lowen and John Pierrakos, whom I'll discuss later, labeled that energy "orgone" or orgasmic energy. Reich believed the pelvic chakra's hourglass was blocked, and saw patients cured of cancer and other serious conditions by helping them move this energy through sluggish bodies by use of an orgone accumulator. Though I'm unsure whether he was exclusively thinking in terms of the energy of physical orgasm when he theorized, he believed "orgasmic" energy, whatever it is, became stuck in the body and actually caused illness. He seemed to affirm the concept that it's impossible to have heart energy, head energy, or gut energy without sacral/sexual energy flow.

Reich's model corresponds nicely to the osteopathic offshoot craniosacral therapy, whose purpose is the enhancement of cerebrospinal fluid and energy movement through the spinal column. This free flow depends entirely on the freedom of movement in the sacrum. So, when we tighten our groin or tuck our tail for any reason, we're slowing our total energy.

I think Reich's main problem was his choice of terminology or "branding." If he'd labeled his "orgasmic" energy with Pierrakos' term "right" energy (Chapter 10) or what I think of as "authentic" energy, he might be a more celebrated pioneer today. He was put in jail by the crusade of an old-fashioned muckraking reporter who objected to discussing sexual energy or the healing benefits of orgasm. No nation should have to stand for such public broadcast of private matters! His detractor won the battle; eventually an assistant misrepresented an orgone accumulator and the federal government shut down all operations. Orgone accumulators were all destroyed and he died in jail in the 1950s just before he was due to be released.

To me we're getting close to a very important concept here. I don't believe one even has to allow physical orgasm to move through their body, if they responsibly find a way to allow shame-free SOAR energy (Sensory, Orgasmic, Authentic, Right (or Reichian) energy—my acronym) to flow and move energy through the sacral chakra. I don't believe orgasm is essential to the flow of this SOAR energy. We just need to shake our tails and let go more often, whether celibate or not. We all could shamelessly allow *some* form of energy to move through the pelvis, and therefore total body, more easily. While sexual energy is important, if celibacy was bad for our health, celibates would be shown statistically to die earlier than actively partnered sexual beings. I don't believe you'd find that result in literature. But unless we move energy, we're dying. Like every mechanical or energetic system, we must keep energy moving to perpetuate the system.

Many of us seem trapped in sexual ambiguity: Am I homosexual, or heterosexual? Where do I fit? It's my belief that if we look at self without shame, we'll find where on the spectrum of homo/bi/heterosex we fit, and allow ourselves to live there. When we allow shame to overtake us, we try to force ourselves to fit on that scale where we believe others want to see us; then try to force others to also fit on our scale. Can we allow ourselves to partner with both our masculine and feminine energies, without worrying that acknowledging our "other" side will make us wrong?

## WHAT DID LOVE LOOK LIKE?

Once we've had an experience, we tend to recreate or duplicate that experience—good or, too often, bad. Here's an interesting train of thought: What did love, or seeming positive energy directed toward you, look and feel like the first time someone shared their sexual energy with you? What happened the first time you realized someone was sending sexual energy your way? Was it a pleasant experience you're trying to duplicate? Did your first sexual energy experience turn into an unpleasant one you're trying to forget, but continue to recreate in your quest to "fix" it? These are important questions if we're serious about freeing sexual energy.

Could it be possible we're trying to coach current partners into duplicating and perhaps repairing our introductions to sexual energy? Many of us still dress emotionally in the old outfit given to us by someone who introduced us, inappropriately, to sex at an early age. If we decided we didn't like this person or what we felt after that initial attention, why do we still wear the garment they put on us? Might we be duplicating unhealthy and stifling feelings of shame each time we engage in or think about sexual activity, just because it's what we first thought it was supposed to be?

One of my mentors, long deceased, said to me, "You know, at some point you have to make up your mind to lose your temper." I've realized that at some point you have to make up your mind to do anything you do, or it never gets done. So you make up your mind whether to allow someone else's behaviors in your early years to control your adult life, or whether to step out of that pattern. You make up your mind to examine the sexual shame you carry from earlier experiences, and decide if it serves you now.

You also make up your mind what kind of sexual commitment you want. Define your needs and set your goals, then choose how and with whom you move sexual energy. Make choices that allow your sexual self to be satisfied. Be comfortable with the primary relationship you've chosen; whether to yourself, a committed partner, a society, or ideal, or who or whatever gets your commitment in the now. If a choice feels uncomfortable, ask yourself why. Keep asking until you drill down to the answers that resolve your conflict.

Choose where, how, and whether you want to move your sexual energy, and do it consciously and deliberately. Then create a space of safety where clients can examine this same choice for themselves. When the question is whether to be sexually active, the choice is simply no or yes. Remember we can be celibate *and* healthy if we find that important SOAR energy. If a person decides to move sexual energy, however, their choices become: self-partnered, committed partners, semi- or uncommitted partnerships, chance encounters, or hired partners (whether in reality or fantasy).

Though I believe one can find depth, meaning, and satisfaction in committed partnership, I can't make that choice for others. I suggest we all examine which place we've chosen and whether that's the place we want to be. Do we thrive and continue to grow? If not, are we ready to make changes? Orgasm for orgasm's sake may move energy and relieve stress, but common sense says orgasm with positive love energy present is healthier than sexual energy movement without love, or with shame.

Like Anna, whether our "down there" is awake or not in our current sexual state, shame over who we are and what we feel isn't required. Too many preachers and teachers try to demand an apology, a denial of self, and acceptance of guilt if we enjoy our sexual feelings or even their possession. If we can't measure up to someone else's sexual standards, perhaps it's time to set reasonable standards for ourselves!

## CREATE WITHOUT SHAME

Sexual organs are second or sacral chakra territory—the area of desire and creation or, conversely, shame. My descriptive phrase for this area is "Responsibly create without shame." Shame rises to judgment (chakra 3) and anchors us in our inadequacies instead of our possibilities. The qualities in a healthy and free second chakra are a relaxed attitude toward sex and survival (a healthy balance of lust/chastity) as well as toward *responsibly* creating and maintaining (sexual and non-sexual) relationships. When guilt and shame close the area, frigidity or inappropriate relationships may occur; an open second chakra allows us to feel, experience, and move sexual energy joyously.

The reproductive system can be seen as both organs and glands: In too many of us, they've lost their vital energy, and our Oriental medicine Lower Burner has nearly lost its fire.

## CORE fascial release of adductor compartment

1. Client on side with knees/hips flexed toward trunk. Pillow for head is fine; bend upper knee in front of lower leg with a pillow under it to get it out of the way. Let the lower leg remain long and straight to access adductor line.

2. Work anywhere up this lower leg to find the tension that seems to often turn the leg in one quarter turn too tight— is the lower leg's heel staying on the table? This is what you'd like to see. Too often it's in the air.

3. From knee to groin, slowly sink into tissue and move across the adductor fibers. As you find a held spot, ask client to move long leg: up toward ceiling, forward away from body, perhaps even asking low back to stay back.

4. Do both legs, even though one seems to be in more trouble. You may find more in front of adductor on one leg and behind adductor on other side.

An important muscle to examine in this chapter is often simply called PC muscle. That's because the scientific name—*pubococcygeus* (from pubic bone to coccyx)—is a bit of a mouthful. We're looking at the musculature that forms the bottom of the pelvis—the pelvic floor (Figure 8.1). Like Anna, many of us store tension here. Others have lost tone entirely. You can imagine why many of us still hold pelvic/ sacral tension and why others have given up their integrity in this charged area. Can we learn to stay relaxed, yet toned? Are genitals and tail tucked tightly to guard against movement and feeling "down there," or do they move easily from a level and living pelvis?

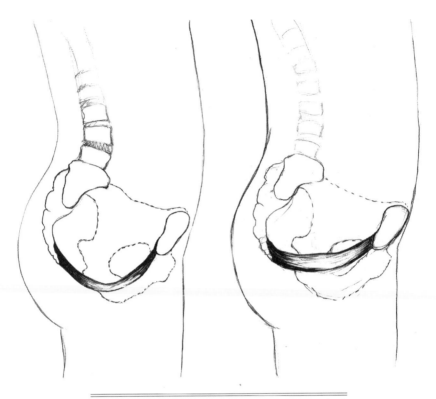

Figure 8.1 PC muscles sagging (L) and toned (R)
*The pelvic floor can be toned or collapsed.*

Another important muscle group to the pelvic floor's operation is the *adductor* compartment, the muscle group on the inside of the legs, into the pelvic floor, which *ad*-ducts or brings the legs together and holds them closed (Figure 8.2). Imagine how someone who's experienced sexual trauma or fear might tighten these muscles to protect their pelvis. Many of us have put a lock and key on the pelvis because we've not been initiated with truly positive sexual touch.

One more important aspect of the pelvic basin…the two rings of pelvic bone we sit on, which are commonly referred to as "sitting bones" instead of *ischial tuberosities* (Figure 8.3). Most of us don't sit equally in these two bones; we place more weight in one or the other, or sit on the front edge of one and the back of the other. Not only should they carry weight equally like feet and legs, we can also intend to stretch them *away from each other*. I sometimes think of the sitting bones as being the feet of the low spine. Do we have a relaxed stance? Do we sit in our heels or toes? Again, as with feet, rocking a bit more to the front lengthens us.

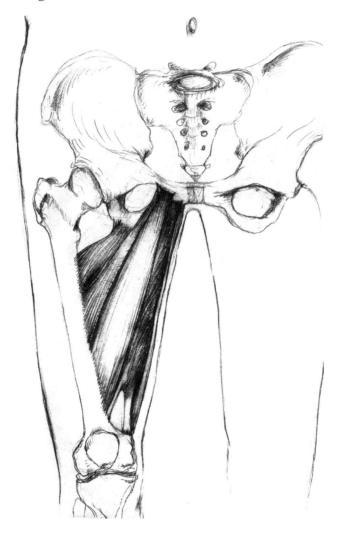

Figure 8.2 Adductor compartment

*Adductors pull the inside of the thigh up and into the
pelvic floor for protection on too many of us.*

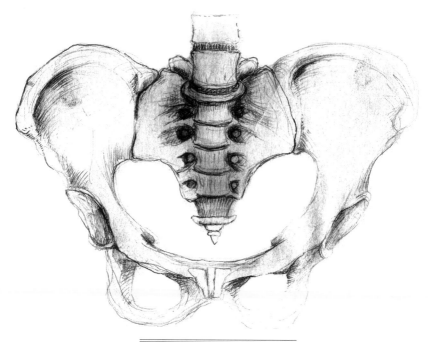

Figure 8.3 Ischial tuberosities
*The ischial tuberosities, or sitting bones, are the feet of
the pelvis: Do you sit on your heels, or your toes?*

Finally, let's add in the sacred or magic triangle—the *sacrum* and its tip, the *coccyx*, as they relate to the insides of both hipbones where they rest, and at the spine, which they support. Does the tail swing freely, or are we like a shamed puppy that's been whipped and tucked his tail between his legs? Does the end of our spine relax, or tighten to further cup, grasp, and choke the pelvis or protect the rectum? Whom do you know who, if quizzed, can't recall at least one tailbone injury?

Move energy! Help clients examine how or when or even whether Sensory Orgasmic Authentic Right energy flows through them. Don't judge their choices about how they share sexual energy, and how deeply they allow self to be moved by it. They must choose how important sex is to them. If it becomes *too* important, they may be moving into dangerous or obsessive behavior, and if they ignore it, they may still live a long and healthy life. But to those who disdain it or are ashamed of it, sickness or unhappiness may come.

## CORE fascial release of tailbone restrictions: Survival and shame

1. Client is prone with feet hanging off the edge of table so that feet are able to flex and extend fully.

2. Look at the heels: Does one heel and leg seem to be pulling tighter, through knee and inner hamstring, into tailbone area? Does the heel actually look shorter and closer to center? There's more work to be done on that side.

3. You may choose to first warm up that side's inner hamstring, and could easily begin the unwinding process at the heel. After hamstring, gently place your finger just to the outside of the coccyx, at the sacrotuberous and ischiococcygeal ligaments. Work to create space—gently!—between these two bones, and ask client to imagine a wagging tail as they breathe and stretch that same side heel as you work. The more the client holds heel long and to the outside, the more they enhance your work.

4. Again, this work is about the client letting go, not about you creating change. Go gently!

5. Side two is usually easier for the client.

As I've challenged myself to learn to stretch any of the body's hinges from any other, I also want to create more simultaneous directions and techniques for you to explore and share with clients. I challenge you to create more of these stretches for yourself and to be more bold in asking clients to examine and deal with their sexual/sacral energy slowdown, as well. It's time to acknowledge and stretch the genitals, without shame.

Perhaps the deepest, yet most subtle, stretch I've found asks the hip hinge and pelvic floor to stretch out of the lumbosacral junction— to access, wake up, feel, and enjoy our pelvises. We've already hinted at this earlier…try it for yourself. Lie on the floor or a bed with knees and legs downlong—pull your navel further back into the surface (straightback), but *imagine* you can also ask your hips and genitals to pull farther away from that back (forwardlongaway). Get your genitals and back farther away from each other. Now, put breath energy into this new space. What feelings come up for you? Are you shamed or embarrassed by them? Relax and be unashamed of your pelvic region.

How do you tone your pelvic bowl? (See Figure 8.4.) Dr. Milton Kegel popularized an exercise which now bears his name. The Kegel exercise is to simply muscularly start and stop the flow during urination. I believe it's important to tone the muscles of the pelvic floor; but I suggest a new concept to this exercise when I ask clients to focus on their feelings of relaxation as well as feelings of tightening. In other words, don't focus just on learning to tighten the bowl. Focus also on allowing the pelvic floor to relax and letting energy flow. And, can you ask for this tightening and release while the low back stays back?

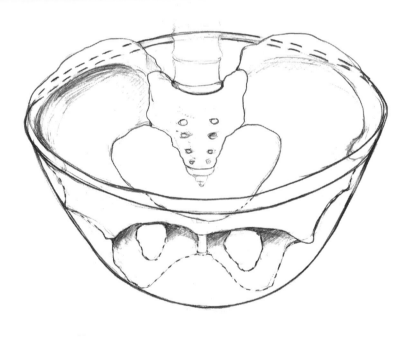

Figure 8.4 Pelvis as a bowl

*Too often we "spill our guts" forward. Can you carry
a level bowl so as to not spill the contents?*

## THE ONE WE'VE GOT

Years ago I taught public school music in a very rural area. One evening I met a new parent, the father to several of my students. What he said to me has stayed for many years: "Mr. Cherry [sic], you may not be the best music teacher in the world, but you're the one we've got."

Was this an insult or a compliment? I truly didn't know. After a bit of reflection the interpretation I chose was, "I don't know anything about you, but you've come here to try to teach my children, so we'll treat you like you're the best music teacher in the world." His kids worked hard for me. They weren't greatly intelligent, but they were good hearted, and always followed rules and requests in my classes. They gave their best to the best music teacher they knew.

That parent's words were a milestone for me. I often remember "I'm the one I've got" and I celebrate that fact. I translate this simple statement into many aspects of my life, including the sexual arena. I may not be the best person in the world, but I'm the one I've got. I may not have the most beautiful body and face in the world, but it's the one I've got. I may not have the most exciting and fulfilled sexual life in the world, but it's the one I've got. I'm grateful for and excited by the one I've got. "I'm enough." Too many people believe physical attractiveness correlates to sexual satisfaction, so they need to attract beauty and be seen as beautiful.

But the trick, the technique that makes life *and* sex joyous, is to decide and believe the one you've got is not only good enough, but that it's satisfying. I encourage my clients to believe they don't have to achieve perfection. In fact, wouldn't perfection either be boring, or very difficult to sustain? We only have to be satisfied with ourselves, with who and what and where we are right now, and with how far we've come—our process and our progress. I invite you to celebrate who and what you are and what you have instead of wishing you could be someone or something else. Enjoy the pelvis without climbing into judgment. Discern what makes you whole.

In *You Can Heal Your Life* (1984) Louise Hay suggests we learn to do mirror work—to be able to look in the mirror and say, truthfully: "I love and approve of myself exactly the way I am." Try speaking that statement to your reflection in the mirror and you'll see it brings up lots of issues! Too many of us can't face ourselves without qualifiers: "...except...but...other than..." Hay challenges us to look into the eyes of the person in the mirror, affirm perfection, and learn to believe in self. We are perfect. We may not resemble the current beautiful models, but we're the perfect us. We *must* learn to celebrate: "We're the ones we've got."

Here's an interesting experiment: Look at your own eyes in a mirror, one eye at a time. Allow the eye you're staring into to become the person who first awakened your sexual feelings. Now change and meet the other eye, maintaining the connection to that initiator. Then, after feeling your feelings, become the person *you* were then, and look at both eyes individually again. What feels damaged in you?

I'm beginning to suggest that clients stretch in front of a mirror. Imagine dressing provocatively, or dressing in comfortable clothing that makes you look and feel good, and stretching in front of a mirror. Imagine taking off clothes to work in front of a mirror. Imagine allowing yourself to feel the movement of sacral and sexual energy while stretching in front of the mirror. Do these imaginings challenge and frighten you?

Refer to Figure 8.5 and say to clients: "Try the adductor stretch shown that invites you to feel the inside of your legs and pelvic floor. As you let your heels slide downout along the wall *while* keeping your low back downback, and neck outlong, imagine allowing your adductor muscles to realize how tight and traumatized they've become. You—more sensibly than anyone—have a key to unlock and unwind these sexual deep lines of holding. Be unashamed."

Find some way to ask yourself, then your clients, to stretch not only body tissues, but also the ego's belief in self-worth, attractiveness, and sexual desirability. We must believe in these attributes personally before others can find them in us. We can turn loose of how we look, or how we should look, as we stretch. We really can't change the basics of the way we look; it's who we're supposed to be. For clients: "Make peace and learn to like yourself as you stretch, sexually. The sooner you can stretch through shame, leading with free and joyous genitals, the more sexual healing you'll find."

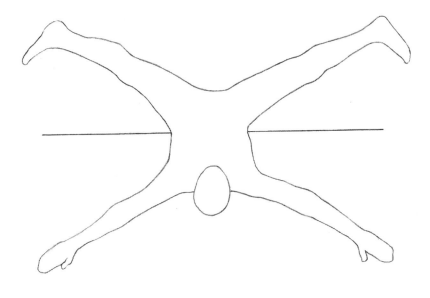

Figure 8.5 Adductor stretch
*The adductor stretch lets you decide how hard to
work your deep line...don't overdo!*

## AS YOU THINK

So much of true sexual health resides in that higher sexual organ—the brain. When we believe we're desirable, we are. Witness how overweight women often find a man who really loves the extra pounds. Witness how very tall or short people often find their perfect partner even though other tall or short friends continue to claim, "There's just no one out there for me." Of course there is! We must simply remove the sign from our forehead that says, "I'm too tall/short/fat/thin, too ugly/poor/stupid. I don't deserve, so I can never have a happy and exciting relationship." What we focus on expands. If we find ourselves to be undesirable, others will support us. And when we realize our own desirability, no one can stop us from celebrating it!

I challenge us all to discern how and why our SOAR energy isn't flowing the way we want; then change. If you choose celibacy, decide how to channel SOAR energy so it still flows through you. If you choose promiscuity, decide how to mindfully accept so much energy from others in your pelvis, and how you'll respond to consequences that will come your way. If you choose a committed partnership, decide how to most fully share and communicate joyful SOAR energy in that commitment. Whatever level of sexual activity you may choose, wherever it fits on the spectrum, learn to enjoy and honor your sexual energy responsibly, yet shamelessly. Then you can guide your clients toward their authentic energy.

We can't, and shouldn't, tell our clients what the healthy flow of SOAR energy in *their* body looks or feels like. We can't tell them they're wrong, unless they're hurting or disrespecting others in their quest for sexual energy flow. It's a choice: not only the method by which we allow our energy to flow or the form it takes, but also with whom we share it. Good health demands we move energy and keep moving it. Sex is a large part of life, and sexual flow creates health. We deserve that flow in our lives.

# Remember

- Most of us are afraid or ashamed of getting to know and feel our pelvic energy. We need to SOAR: to allow **S**ensory, **O**rgasmic, **A**uthentic, **R**ight energy to move through us. Celebrate who and what you are, sexually, without shame or guilt!

- Our first sexual stirrings, whether invited by us or forced upon us, may shape the way we experience sexual touch today. How or even whether to move sexual energy through the body is now a personal decision.

- Learning to create and occupy space between the low back hinge and the pelvic floor or hip hinge is a key to finding and feeling pelvic energy.

- The higher sex organ is the brain. Remember, as we think, so we are. Without judging self, we must discern what's right for us sexually.

# All purpose cue

"In addition to practicing the Kegel exercises mentioned that focus on tightening and releasing the pelvic floor, begin to allow yourself to look at, feel, and breathe your body 'down there.'"

# Client challenge

### EASY

Stand: Sink your inner arches floordown *while* you relax your inner knees and pull your low back upback out of your groin. Allow yourself to feel your sexual/sacral energy without judging it.

### MEDIUM

Bend forward, keeping the back longupback. Allow the fingertips, knuckles, or even palms to touch the floor. Pull your anus upback *while* you reach downfront with your head *while* you sink into your inner arches. Move softly! Only go as far as your body will let you go. Focus first on the feeling of stretch in the back of your legs; then move up to your hips, genitals, and low back. Can you pull your genitals out of your adductors while your inner arches stay anchored? Remember to breathe!

### DIFFICULT

Stand straight with hands on the back of the head and elbows skyup. Now form your body into a forward C curve—thrust with your navel, then make a half circle from side to front to second side. When you've explored this half circle, find more penmanship directions and spots to stretch. Then move down the body slightly and ask the genitals to lead this forward thrust. Focus on pulling one elbow skyup and the same side testis/ovary downlong on first one side, then the other, *both* out of your waist. Now, lead with the head instead of elbows: pull your head upoutside of your testicle or ovary on one side, then the other.

## INTRIGUING

If you're used to flaunting your sexuality, focus on a different chakra. If you're used to hiding your sexuality, experiment with allowing it to arrive first. Allow yourself to have loving feelings for the person you see in the mirror.

## IMAGINE

As you stand or sit to urinate, which foot or sitting bone (depending on your posture) carries more of your weight? Which part of the foot or sitting bone connects (inside, outside, front, or back)? What happens if you shift to the other side of the body? Does it feel very foreign, even difficult? Further, can you hold your low back back while urinating?

# CHAPTER 9

# RELAX THE LOINS

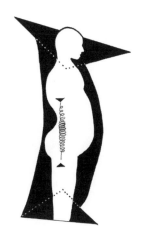

## STEADY ON—LOCKED, OR LOOSE?

*Simply put, we lock our knees, tuck our tails, and gird our loins to cope.*

Helen started me thinking about how we hold on to coping mechanisms and build defenses beyond their immediate usefulness. At session three or four of a ten-session series of Structural Integration, Helen asked, "Did you notice I didn't have my hand on the wall today when we talked?" I had to admit, I was neither aware that her hand wasn't on the wall or that it'd been there when we'd talked previously. She proceeded to explain.

She'd grown up with verbally and emotionally abusive parents. After her father was killed tragically when she was about eight, her mother became even angrier, and poured that bitterness into her child. Helen has distinct memories of both parents berating her, and of creating a solution—a personal talisman.

Whenever she entered a room with either parent in it, she'd immediately place her hand on a wall. As she explained to me: "The wall was my safety. I felt as long as I could touch a wall anything they said or did went right through me and into it. That way I never had that stuff stuck in me." This young child perfected a skill to survive the ugliness life tossed at her. She intuitively understood energetic flow and consciously refused to accept or anchor the unresolved thought forms of others.

A pretty amazing solution for a young child, isn't it? At 45, Helen was finally letting go of the wall. She'd used it for all those years as a survival mechanism, but it was no longer appropriate, so she came to me for help in breaking old physical patterns. At the same time, she worked through outdated emotional baggage with a psychiatrist. When she chose to release her past, the somatopsychic coping skill of anchoring to the wall left her. She discarded the too-small and outdated clothing of that abused child.

And yet…Helen's body held a great deal of physical tension, which seemed to me to be centered from her knees to stomach. I felt she was pulling the essence and energy of her being up into her loins; in doing so, she tightened her knees so severely that they hurt. There was no shock absorbency in her knees because they were constantly pulled into her CORE to protect her. As there had been sexual abuse in her past there were clearly second chakra issues, but also in the loins, knees to pelvis, and into her back. Survival is served by all the loins, chakras 1–3. Let's dig a bit further as we relax our knees out of our fears.

In Chapter 5 on feet I suggested many of us are afraid to touch the ground. This tension may manifest as high arches in the feet and lack of energy to the toes, but many are too tight from knees to loins. Our "survive without fear" and "create without shame" chakras are tightened; our *femoral*, or thigh, arteries and nerves are choked; we have no energy to legs, knees, or feet.

Knees represent flexibility, adaptability, and shock absorbency when they're working properly. When we unlock our knees, we create resilience through the core of our being. When they lock, we brace against the world. As knees soften we allow the tail to loosen and lengthen in a way that further unwinds the core. As we use our knees and tail flexibly instead of tightly, we again enhance blood and cerebrospinal fluid movement through the spine. We oil our brains and our nervous system by loosening our tails and relaxing our knees. As we find flexibility, we're even on a road to healing some of our own nervous disorders.

## IT'S THE KIDNEYS!

Do you wonder what early conditions or situations made people choose their current defense/survival patterns? What makes one person "weak in the knees" while another locks down? What makes someone a "tightass" while someone else is a "pushover"? Issues from feet to pelvis are governed by that base of the spine. As we turn loose of control and believe in our security, we firmly plant and relax. Doesn't it make sense that the more we can flexibly plant feet, yet soften knees, the more we relax our pelvic floor? And as we soften, I believe we're allowing our kidneys to more fully process the negativity from our bodymindcores.

In classical Oriental medicine kidneys are the ultimate bringer of health. As kidneys weaken, we age. If kidneys can't process or eliminate waste and negative energy, we speed our demise. Isn't it interesting that the Kidney *meridian* (which isn't meant to be confused with the kidney *organ*, which, while on the meridian, doesn't rule the line) begins at the big toe and goes up the inside of the leg in the adductors? From here, pick up the Heart/Uterus meridian (*ban mao*) and/or the Central Channel (*chun mai*), deeply, and we're in the belly, along the front of the spine, at the psoas, iliacus, and quadratus lumborum, which last is becoming a new favorite of mine to release the back, shoulders, and knees. And remember my interest in adrenals in Chapter 1? They rest on the kidneys, on top of this loin line.

For the client (and you): "What happens if you ground yourself in your feet, hold arches into the floor, flex knees, soften your deep line, and draw circles, eights, lines, or crescents with the knees *while* the arches remain grounded? Do you feel vulnerable if you keep your low back upback *while* you're pushing arches to the floor *while* you draw the circles or other patterns with the knees?" Too many of us think we have "bad" knees—weak, arthritic, or damaged. Many of us don't let knees perform their shock absorbing job. The old saying "use it or lose it" has been proved true for too many of us.

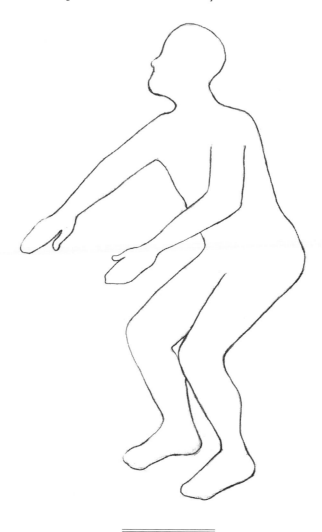

Figure 9.1 Squats
*Simple squats can bring life to knees, hips, ankles, and toes.*

I suggest clients try a few mild knee bends (Figure 9.1). "Do your knees talk to you and ask you to stop? Many of us can barely squat, yet some cultures live much of their lives in a squatting position and have far fewer physical problems in their bodies. What would life be like if we could learn to use 'knee push ups,' simply bending and squatting mildly while the feet stay anchored on the ground, or while we push up through the toes?" Wouldn't this action oil the knees and move energy through them to strengthen the shock absorbency of the entire body? What would happen if we allowed ourselves to sink into and *through* the knees, ankles, and toes with each step forward?

## STAND YOUR GROUND—SAFELY

If my goal is flexible knees, I can take steps to meeting this goal when I let myself go up or down stairs while tracking both feet straight ahead. While keeping my body in an upright posture I can let my weight sink through parts of my toes that don't like connecting with the step's surface: inner, outer—even the tip of the big toe can take the stress of a foot ascending or descending a step. When I allow the front and inner foot to bear the *weight* and *wait*, then sink into the stretch, allowing the big toe to *be long* and *belong*, change finds me. Everything changes when one climbs or descends steps with feet pointed straight ahead! As I work both toe and knee hinge, every part of my body seems to be getting a deep line workout. Lately I've even tried to shift my weight to various parts of the foot like a surfer or a tango dancer might do.

Remember, my ultimate goal with sinking, squatting, and knee bending is farther up the line in the loins. I'm specifically interested in two muscles—the first just inside the hipbones is the *iliacus* (Figure 9.2). I feel if and when we learn to relax this muscle, we've finally unwound our loins. Too many of us hold our breath and tighten our legs up into our spine and ribcage, through the hipbone and on into the muscle on top of it, the *quadratus lumborum*, which reaches all the way to the spine and the last rib (Figure 9.3). These two taken together, I call *ilioquadratus*; to me they *are* the "gird your loins" muscle. They make us tighten the inside of the leg up into the back to survive whatever comes. They help me visualize how important soft knees are to free hips and a loose tail.

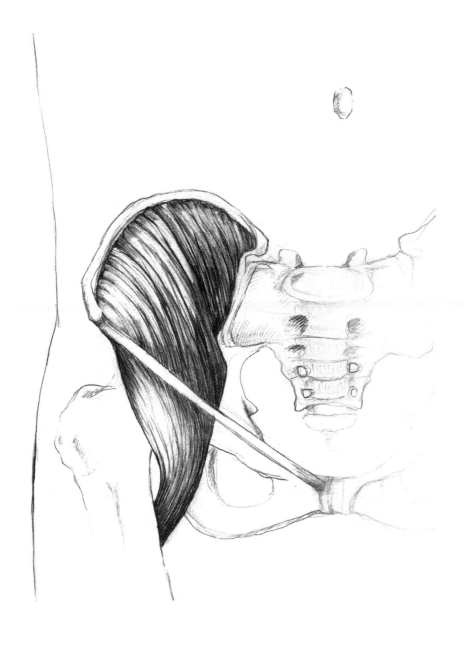

Figure 9.2 Iliacus muscle

*Imagine the hipbone as a spoon; this muscle covers the interior
and goes to the lesser trochanter where it joins the psoas.*

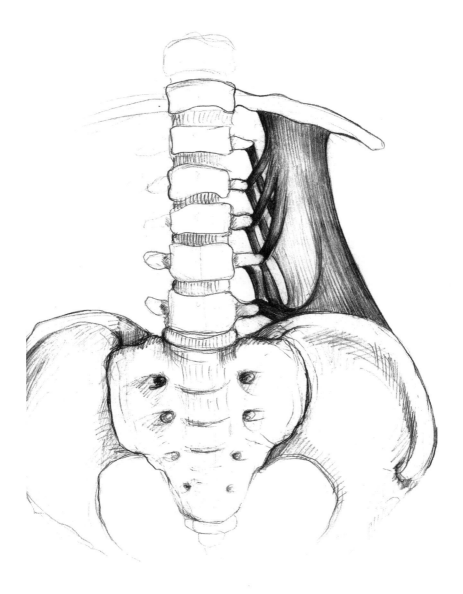

Figure 9.3 Quadratus lumborum

*This muscle runs from the crest of the ilium to the 12th rib, but also attaches to the back, outside, and front of distal transverse processes. Consider it and the iliacus as one muscle with a hipbone spacer: ilioquadratus, the "gird your loins" muscle.*

## CORE fascial release of quadratus lumborum and iliacus: Ungird

1. Quadratus: Client on side. Sit or kneel, pointed toward client's head, on table/couch, with your hip touching client hip/low back. Allow elbow to rest on their superior ASIS line. With your elbow, follow this line toward the erectors, staying anchored on the crest of hipbone, not the ribs! Client breath is always important. Let your touch be down toward the floor, but glancing off the hip, away from client, towards yourself.

2. If this is too difficult or uncomfortable for either of you (and if you're honest, you'll know whether you're following intention or ego), place client prone with feet off edge, as for tailbone work. Place a forearm in the quadratus area, just above crest of hip. Move across—in or out, but always lightly across tissue while client lengthens same leg and turns heel in and out...and breathes. Real change.

3. Iliacus tightens deep line to the feet, high arches, and even bunions! Client is supine; imagine the iliacus as a spoon that you want to clean out. Work slowly inside hipbone toward the lower iliacus attachment while client pulls same side foot/heel/inner arch as far from your fingers as possible. You don't need to move far or deep to make a change. This connection surprises most clients.

I don't think there's a magic bullet to make everyone better, which is why I've included so many stretches along with techniques. But I've long known that success in the knees comes from ankles and especially from hips and the low back. The adductor release from the previous chapter often helps to soften knees too. We've worked with feet, hips/tail, and guts; so let's continue that line into the loins, realizing we're working near and on the kidneys. Think again of holding the waist back: Do you see how this tones the kidneys and invites healthy flow?

Many of us jam one leg into its hip more than the other—chiropractors often tell patients they have one leg shorter. I believe they have one hip higher/tighter. A simple awareness can help clients change this configuration: "Lie down and pull one heel/inner arch as far from your hips as you can. At the same time, jam the other heel and straight leg up into your pelvis as tightly as you can. Hold this position and breathe several times (Figure 9.4). Relax for a moment; then change the direction so the tightened leg becomes the long one and the longer leg now shortens. Chances are in one side you'll find a bit more tension as you stretch." I'm finding many clients with sciatic pain can keep their problem at bay with this simple stretch.

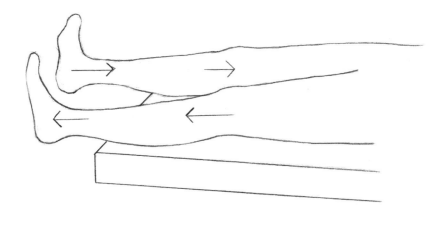

Figure 9.4 Sacroiliac stretch

*Jam one leg into the pelvis while pulling the other long and out.*

I'm getting intrigued by the relationships of *sacroiliac* (SI) junctions, right and left, and the *lumbosacral* junction at the top of the sacrum: a "magic" triangle (Figure 9.5). Common sense tells me we need balance in this triangle; yet I find most of us jammed too tightly in one side or the other. What might be too tight? Many things, but...if you've tried tailbone and adductor work already, next look to the iliacus, quadratus, and psoas; then the erectors, latissimus, and obliques; next think of the tensor fascia lata and the iliotibial band, hamstrings, and quadriceps. The previous stretch may help the client identify what's holding as it clears and balances the area. Pulling the legs and SI joints long *while* pulling the head long allows us to again stretch two ends of our rubber band.

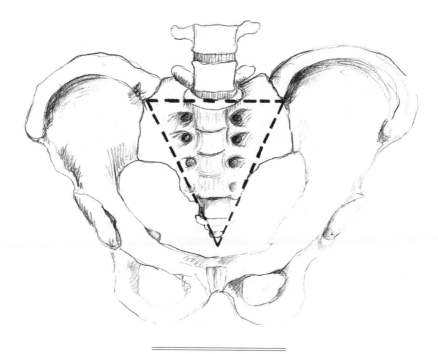

Figure 9.5 Magic triangle
*Can we create equality in the two SI joints?*

Remember that coccyx: Like a puppy dog waiting to be punished, we've tucked and tightened our tail against the impending blow (which may have come and gone long ago). Simply softening the loins, believing in the surety of our survival, and moving as if it's all right for the tail to swing can begin to change hard mental attitudes that tighten physical tissues. You're surviving, and thriving! Wag your tail!

## HOW WE CONGEST AND HOW WE COPE

Our congestors, the stuck stimulus or unresolved thought forms, may come from outside us as a physical, emotional, mental, chemical, or energetic trauma. We're in charge of how we perceive and process that stimulation or thought form. We can suffer a physical insult, be sickened by emotional pain, or get mentally overscheduled and overstimulated. Chemicals congest us: Drug or alcohol dependency, overuse of caffeine or sugar, toxic foods, and environmental poisoning slow our energies. We can be congested by outside energies such as power lines, fluorescent lights, cell phones, and even noise. Any of these stimuli can shorten our deep line and cause us to tighten our loins.

We're bombarded with countless messages that slow down or stop the flow of energy through our bodies and minds. Our coping mechanisms placate, dilute, and accommodate these outside influences instead of sorting, processing, and releasing them. Simply put, we lock our knees, tuck our tails, and gird our loins to cope. Eventually these coping behaviors slow down our energetic bodymindcores even more. Coping mechanisms may have helped us through earlier times, but now it's good to ask if these skills are still needed.

## A FRIENDLY UNIVERSE?

As a thinker, few have paralleled Albert Einstein, who I mentioned earlier had decided to live in a friendly universe. If Einstein believed in the benevolence of the Universe, why can't I believe also? Why shouldn't I act as if the Universe wants to reward me richly, and the only thing that gets in its way is me? Why don't I believe the Universe is a safe and secure place where I can happily plant my feet, soften my knees, and wag my tail?

We speed our demise by driving our trauma in ever deeper and, like Helen, hanging onto our personal wall with all our might. So challenge clients to inventory old coping patterns: "Look at the old costumes you've worn…why are they still here? Are they appropriate? Have you gotten bigger? Did the seasons pass them by? Do you have different tastes? Do you have any idea why you chose them in the first place? Stop coping and defending; throw away what's no longer working for you. Make room for greater good in your life by taking your hand off the wall and unlocking your knees."

Remember, clients are sensitive. If you choose to ungird loins on others, you'd better have done your work too!

# Remember

- We all have old coping skills that cause us to hold our breath, harden our hearts, stand our ground, and gird our loins. These behaviors may no longer be necessary or useful, if the ground below us is stable. Is it?

- Too many of us forget the knees should serve as a resilient shock absorber for the deep line which allows energy to move through the body—we're shortening ourselves to the kidneys with every step instead of flowing through life. We gird our loins.

- A stimulus or thought form comes at us from the outside world; but we're in charge of how we perceive, process, and respond to that stimulus—or how we store it in our body.

## All purpose cue

"As you're standing, sink and anchor into the ground, allowing the deep line of your body to relax. Bring your pelvis forward and your low back farther back *while* your feet stay anchored into the ground, your knees stay soft, and your hips lengthen out of your back. Now, think 'safety.' Does this feel different to you? Practice finding this place and operating from it. Imagine the crests of your hipbones can stay level and tall *while* your knees sink away from them to the ground."

## Client challenge

### Easy

As you stand, find your tailbone. Let it hang (think wag) as you sink your feet and legs floordown out of it *while* you lift your ribcage and head skyup out of it.

## MEDIUM

Lie on your back. As you tune into your body, do you feel one hip living higher off the ground than the other? Cross your legs, with the *lower* hip's ankle crossing over the higher hip's knee. Now pull that high hip's knee to the midline *while* the high hip pushes itself downback into the floor.

## DIFFICULT

Stand with your belly button backupback while you ask the crotch to stay forwarddown. Now, undulate hips side to side while holding length between the crotch and midback. Breathe.

## INTRIGUING

Think about the muscular action of standing still. Can you realize there's no such thing as standing still? Allow yourself to exaggerate circles or back and forth movements that let all parts of the foot touch the ground, as you work to create balance and resilience above.

## IMAGINE

It may be time to return to reflexology on self or clients: Sometimes, entering the central channel or CORE line through the feet, specifically the stomach and costal arch points, occiput, shoulders, or anywhere on the spine, will allow a tight and bound person to unwind deeply.

# CHAPTER 10

# LEAD WITH YOUR HEART

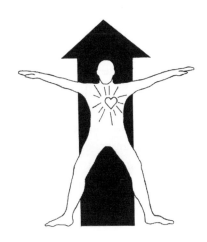

## THE CORE BLOOM—BARREN, OR FULL?

*When we're on purpose, when "our heart's in it," life is lived enthusiastically. If our heart's not in it, life is just endured.*

Naomi was an early client of mine who represents many of us; a beautiful young person so stooped forward that she appeared not only to be much older and shorter than she actually was, but she seemed to have no chest. Naomi's work made her sit at a computer all day. She loved her work, but she couldn't stand upright. After an early session, I advised Naomi she might want to experiment in her world "leading with her heart." Immediately she burst into tears and said, "I could never do that."

Too many of us are afraid of our heart, our CORE muscle, our essence. Can we learn to let our hearts stay open to not only the happy and loving stimuli that come our way, but also to the fearful or angry energy that often tries to penetrate and perhaps overwhelm us? Let's remove barriers and let SOAR energy flow into us *while* we learn how to let it flow *through* and out of us. When we open the heart, breathe, and allow energetic flow, life is good. We're satisfied with our progress and our process.

The heart center is key: this middle, first of the upper chakras, is also the middle dantian center and Emperor of the Chinese body, responsible for the free working of the heart, circulatory system, and the *thymus* gland, which regulates overall body energy. Consider, this burner space is also connected directly to the first/second chakras by the Heart/Uterus meridian and the Central Channel. Emotionally the heart is meant to express joy and compassion as we take up space: too many of us close off these emotions and live with a shielded heart in the "cardinal sin" of envy or competition, developing a lordotic posture that rigidly withstands any challenge. Others oversubmit to the virtue, kindness, and kyphosis. Either way, the heart and back suffer. Words I use to describe an open heart chakra are "Enthusiastically quest without yearning." Yearning rules when we're not doing what we want to do, on purpose. When we turn loose of our need to defeat others to gain our desires and live in enthusiastic satisfaction, we're living from the heart.

When we're on purpose, when "our heart's in it," life is lived enthusiastically. If our heart's not in it, life is just endured. The fields of pop psychology and self-help are filled to overflowing with books that tell you how to live a fuller, happier, purposeful, prosperous life. Being on purpose helps one get up with enthusiasm and go to bed with a feeling of accomplishment. Many studies have shown that happy and purpose-driven people live longer.

To some degree we all get demoralized in our lives, and need something or someone—some purpose—to keep our morale strong. We live, or die, on purpose. Do you know the story of Viktor Frankl? A student of Sigmund Freud and a Jew, Frankl was incarcerated in a concentration camp during the Second World War. As a psychologist, he chose to fill his time in the camp studying fellow prisoners. He began to notice some prisoners remained healthy under horrible circumstances, while others withered and died. He observed that those who found a purpose for survival, a positive *or* negative reason to drive them, managed to stay alive. Frankl tells his story in *Man's Search for Meaning* (1959). His message is simply, those who live on purpose, live longer. Are we allowing ourselves to put heart into our lives and life into our hearts?

## VITAMIN "G"

What we focus on expands. When we focus on how tired and miserable we are, it will be more so. If we focus on how happy and wealthy and grateful we are, it will be more so. When we focus on feelings of joy, compassion, and openness in our heart area, we'll grow them. When we know what or who it is we want to be, feel the condition we want, and give thanks for all that is, we magnetize good to our heart.

Jerome Frank says in his book *Persuasion and Healing* (Frank and Frank 1961) that we become ill when we're demoralized. It follows that the role of the therapist is to try to help clients become *re-moraleized* (my word)—to find their purpose, meaning, and gratitude for life. I don't consider myself to be a nutritionist; I barely remember to take my few vitamins each day. Clients often want me to suggest what they should take to improve their digestion, circulation, bone strength, etc. My short answer is: I have no idea.

My longer answer is a bit intriguing. I really believe whatever we ingest has nutrition in it if we could be grateful for that which comes at us! While there are clearly better and worse foods (and emotions), if we can be grateful for *whatever* comes our way (be it food, emotions, actions from others, or the Universe) and seek to absorb the nutrition from the experience and eliminate the garbage, we're taking in Vitamin "G." We'll more fully receive our appropriate and needed nutrition. When we mindlessly, dutifully, achingly stuff our faces and souls with toxic emotions and foods to dilute our heartaches, we're bound to suffer from an overdose of Vitamin B negative. My personal diet (physical or emotional) isn't pure, but I feed on gratitude much more frequently than negativity. Too many of us try to survive on mega-doses of toxic emotions.

## THE CENTER OF RIGHT ENERGY

I like the "Center Of Right Energy" as an acronym for CORE. The phrase was coined by John Pierrakos, founder of the CORE Energetics technique and author of *CORE Energetics: Developing the Capacity to Love and Heal* (2005). Pierrakos expanded his mentor Wilhelm Reich's orgone energy work (see Chapter 8) and with colleague Alexander Lowen refined it into the "body armor" freeing technique they named "Bioenergetics." Pierrakos evolved his techniques further, incorporated his wife Eva's ideas, and began practicing and teaching CORE Energetics.

In my interpretation of Pierrakos' work, each of us is a three-layered being. The deep layer is his CORE or Center Of Right Energy. It's what I think of as the essence of the person—the center of authentic energy, located in or near the heart. The next layer of being is the Body, and the third layer is our Environment. Too many of us lock our center of right energy *inside* that body layer and don't allow any permeation or communication between core and environment (cold hands, warm heart). In a healthy bodymindcore, we bring the environment into the core happily and fearlessly. Oriental medicine also teaches that our inability to exchange energy with our environment causes our dis-ease. Some of us never move easily from layer to layer. We protect the core tightly with the body to keep the center of right energy from experiencing our outer world. We hold our breath if we send the heart out into the world, expecting it to be hurt.

I see this core essence enclosed in a tight fist or box at the center of our being, roughly behind our sternum and in front of our heart. Recall how the diaphragm's hiatuses or openings allow energy and fuel through the umbrella. The sternum or breastbone acts as the body layer/shield which covers and protects both heart and CORE. Much of the work I do encourages clients to let go of the tension in this deep "essence" spot. Doesn't it make sense that releasing core tension allows energy to flow more smoothly throughout the body's systems, since the heart pumps blood to every other part of the body? Too many of us tighten the heart area: "congestive" heart failure, high or low blood pressure, aneurisms or weakening of blood vessel walls, valve problems, heart attacks; all come when the heart is unhappy, weak, and tight, not resilient.

## CONGESTION VS CIRCULATION

Why do I spend so much time in a chapter supposedly devoted to the heart talking about gratitude, purpose, and CORE essence? Because, I believe too many of us are like Naomi: The slowdown of energy caused by unprocessed, unfulfilled, ungrateful thoughts and feelings or shortened postures contributes greatly to problems in the area of the heart.

Therapist: Stand for a moment. Thrust your pelvis forward and out as we've done previously. Lift your head upback again as your waist also stays level. Hold this posture and pushlift your heart upfront *while* you pull your diaphragm down. How does this feel? Can you take up heartspace, or must you retreat?

We sometimes forget the heart is a muscle *and* organ as well as a chakra. Its aorta or central distribution channel carries oxygenated blood from the heart to the arteries and down through the capillaries, where this rich fuel contacts and nourishes every cell of the body (Figure 10.1). After feeding the various body parts, blood returns cellular waste products to the lungs through the venules and veins. Then it's processed, cleaned, and re-oxygenated in the lungs, and returns to the heart again to begin the circuit once more—for thousands of times each day. So the heart's not just a muscle; it's the most important, constantly working muscle in the body. No wonder the Chinese call it Emperor!

The heart rests on top of the diaphragm, anchored in *pericardial* tissue. Tightening this tissue through mental or physical habit puts extra strain on the heart. As we shorten and tighten the front of our body, we stop the flow of energy through the heart, decrease the blood circulation through the body, the amount of oxygen in the blood, and the energy we have for life. When our "heart's not in it" and we tighten our core, we're dying more quickly.

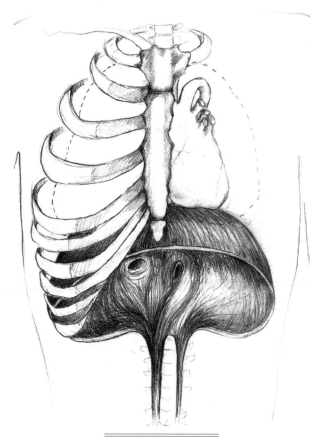

Figure 10.1 The heart
*An organ, hinge, chakra, and Oriental medicine's Emperor.*

Studies abound that show we can regulate our heart's beating and the pressure at which our blood flows. Many of these studies show that relaxation, meditation, tai chi, biofeedback, or some form of calming the mind will soothe the body and enhance overall well-being. In other words, when we're in a relaxed process, our heart muscle can work happily and appropriately.

Let's encourage clients to exercise the heart for resilience/ strength instead of tension/strength. This can be done through cardio strengthening exercise, and I highly recommend we all exert ourselves wisely at least every other day to exercise the circulatory system and heart. Personally I believe nothing serves the entire being or enhances the body experience better than a brisk walk or activity where we truly focus on enjoying the way our body moves. Conversely, a walk that's being taken because one must achieve five miles in an aching body probably doesn't help the heart or the body much.

## THE HEART HINGE

How do we open our hearts? Recall my hourglass image from Chapter 3 and the diaphragm release work we did there (Figure 10.2). This is still my most effective heart work. Common sense suggests we learn to keep this "heart hinge" or heart chakra area open to allow blood, circulation, nerve impulse, lymph, qi, prana, SOAR, or whichever word you might prefer to call energy to travel through the body. For a quarter century I've been challenging clients to open their heart hinge.

### CORE fascial release of the heart (from the back): Turtle

1. Client is prone. Feet on table are fine; face in cradle is all right, but it's better to have them face down in the table with feet off edge if you can only have one or the other.

2. Find the most prominent outward curvature of their spine, which is often in the thoracic range from T4 to 8. This is where too many of us close our heart hinge.

3. Apply mild forearm pressure on one side's erectors; take that pressure laterally in either direction instead of down into the body.

4. Ask client to move into a cobra-like posture of lifting back of head and neck longup (think of a turtle's neck), while you anchor on the stuck spot, while they breathe. Then ask them to move into somersault position with tucked chin and C 4 or 5 vertebra pushing toward ceiling. Make sure the low back doesn't shorten and tighten as you work on the mid and upper back.

5. Use where needed to open any stuck hinge, especially in the heart area.

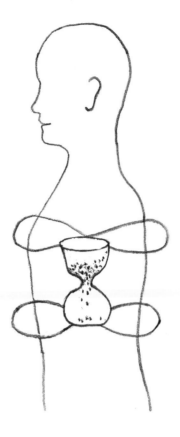

Figure 10.2 Hourglass again

*If energy gets stuck at the psoas/diaphragm, the upper and lower body can't communicate or circulate.*

For some of us, work requires us to bend forward as a computer operator, hairdresser, artist, massager, or a driver might do. For others it's a totally different, emotional cause: We believe that by bending forward and closing off the heart area we make a smaller target for those "bad" things: the negative thought forms, the slings and arrows life shoots at us (Figure 10.3).

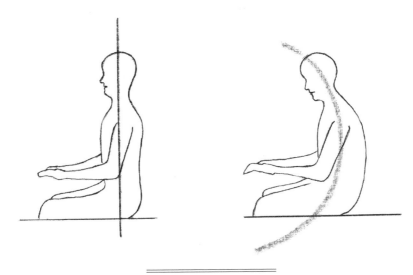

**Figure 10.3 Slump again**
*Can you see how a slumping posture puts undue
pressure on the heart hinge and aorta?*

Some of us are so demoralized we simply don't want to take up space. Think of a pre-teen girl who gets her growth spurt ahead of her friends. As she develops the first breasts among her group, won't she feel awkward? What does she do? She tries to shrink and collapse forward to fit her group. She hides her heart. Think of an abused young person who now faces the world in a tight, angry body. How can they express heart energy? For too many reasons, too many of us practice closing off this heart hinge area, and it's killing us.

In addition to bodywork technique, sometimes I can help clients open their heart hinge area simply by suggesting they lie on the floor with a pillow, bolster, ball, or other object under their heart area that "pops" them forward and open (Figure 10.4). As they remember to breathe (remember to breathe?), relax, and soften, they'll eventually find the connective tissue in their shortened and tightened body wants to release and allow them to stand and sit tall. Often they also find that emotionally they feel more open and secure; it feels safe to keep the heart open.

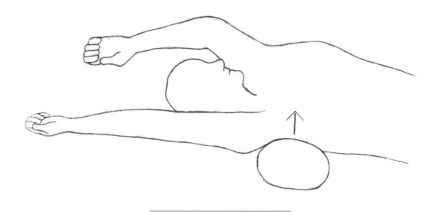

Figure 10.4 Using a bolster

*Any bolster can encourage the heart hinge to remain more open.*

I occasionally suggest clients like Naomi could "lead with their heart" as they go back into the world. Many tell me they couldn't possibly be that vulnerable. When this fear response comes from a client, I'll further suggest they put a mirrored shield or filter over their heart when they feel unsafe; that way whatever comes at them from their environment can be sent right back to its source until they feel strong enough to deal with it. Usually this image allows them to experiment with remaining open to concentrate on creating postural, emotional, and energetic space.

Only when we find and honor our purpose can we live the life we're destined to live. When we wear our heart on our sleeve and everywhere in our body; when we slow down and accept with gratitude everything that comes to us, we'll begin receiving ever-more-gratitude-inspiring feelings, thoughts, and gifts. When we give up envy and practice kindness; when we stretch the tissue around our heart and allow ourselves to take up space, we present a bigger target to the world *and* a greater opportunity to accept good in our lives. How do you serve? How do you want to serve? Expect joy and make it happen.

# Remember

- When we're living on purpose, enthusiastically, our heart is already healthier and happier. What you focus on expands. Where do you put your thoughts? Do you feed on "Vitamin B negative," or "Vitamin G"?

- When we find gratitude for what we have and where we are, we're allowing energy to flow more freely through our hearts and bodymindcores. When we allow ourselves to posturally "lead with our heart" we're creating health.

- Too many of us try to protect our CORE and our heart from our *environment* by tightening our *bodies*. Energy must flow between these three layers for true health.

- Remember, the heart organ, chakra, Emperor, and hinge is also a muscle and the giver of life; if we overwork or overtighten it, we'll wear it out. Are you hardening your heart or taking it for a ride?

# All purpose cue

Sitting or standing: "Allow yourself to lead with your heart. Remember your head is the general who sits at the top of the hill and watches the battle below. Let your heart lead the quest and arrive in every situation first." For some of us, this is a very scary proposition. Retreat without shame is an option, but know that looking for good allows us to find it.

# Client challenge

### EASY

Sit, and allow yourself to sink into and slightly in front of the sitting bones. Pull your heart and ribcage up and forward; then pull your head and shoulders upback. Could you learn to enjoy this posture?

## MEDIUM

Stand. Bring the nipples and heart upright, the tail earthdown. Take the elbows or wrists skyup out of the heart, yet keep the head and tail long too. Then learn to move, undulate, and draw penmanship lines with your heart. Keep your weight evenly in the toes *while* you pull your heart up and out.

## DIFFICULT

Stand in a doorway, though standing under a deck that allows you to hang will give you a sturdier platform for this exercise. Place your hands/fingertips on the trim at the top (you may need a stool or boost to reach the trim or deck). While hanging, allow your armpits to stretch upback as you settle/lengthen the entire spine; now collapsing your knees, sink/roll forward and back into your big toes as your back settles downlong. Slowly, shift through various points in your feet and toes; finally into the inner arch of the feet. As you experiment with feeling your feet, let your back relax; hang, absorb the slack between the toes and armpits; then push your heart area upfront, and breathe. Notice your feelings as you anchor in your toes and pull both ends of your body out of your heart hinge.

## INTRIGUING

The next time someone scolds or is angry with you, work to hear them with an open heart.

## IMAGINE

Have a "heart to heart" talk in your head with someone with whom you feel conflicted.

# CHAPTER 11

# FIND YOUR VOICE

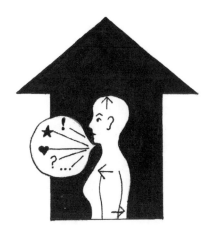

## YOUR EXPRESSION—STRAINED, OR SOARING?

*How have you stopped your own good from flowing through your bodymindcore? Put that question into your own words, and express your truth.*

As we've added layers in each chapter, breathing and stretching, opening spinal curves, grounding into the earth, and leading with the heart, chances are you have trouble doing all these things at once. So will your clients! Yet when we get our three dantian centers (chakras 3/4/6) well spaced, with the waist longback, heart outfront, and head upback, I believe we free our fifth chakra: the throat.

I immediately think of my client Rita in this chapter. A victim of childhood sexual abuse, Rita has suffered from throat issues all of her adult life. After a particularly powerful session of jaw work, she was extremely sick and in bed for a week, until one day, out of the blue, she blurted out: "No, Father, you can't be inside my body anymore!" As soon as she expressed her anger, the throat pain she'd had for years disappeared. She had dealt with eating disorders, addictive behavior, and general unhappiness with her life; after expressing herself, major changes occurred.

This neck center affects the throat, trachea, and esophagus, cervical vertebrae, the *brachial* plexus or nerve and blood network to the arms, and the *thyroid* gland, which is the regulator of energy flowing through the body. When the thyroid shuts down due to blockage in the line from the head to heart to gut, energy through the body slows drastically. Isn't it common sense we'll create more throat energy by lifting our head out of guts and heart? And if we open our throat, won't our ability to express be enhanced? An open throat chakra allows us to "sing" our creativity.

To describe chakra 5, I like the phrase "Freely express without censorship." Censorship suggests the line between the discerning/ judging mechanism in our gut and the worrying/thinking mechanism in our head is clogged. We're weary at the heart and close the throat because we have nothing good to say. I see the cardinal sin/virtue of gluttony/temperance relating to this chakra: not only because we eat and drink to excess, but because we become inappropriately gluttonous or temperate with our expression of feelings.

Visualize a line connecting the gut, heart, and head. Since tugging these three centers together shortens the front of the body and buries the heart farther back, can we choose to lift the head up and heart outfront to allow an open throat? As you try this simple stretch, do you feel an emotional shift? Conditions which might be served by opening the throat center might include throat and thyroid issues, but also neck pain, headaches, TMJ (temporomandibular joint) issues, esophageal problems, and speech difficulties. We've heard of people who have their "heart in their throat," but I'd suggest some of us bury our tongues and our expression down in our hearts.

Most therapists realize the importance of the neck and jaw. I'd like to challenge us to take a deeper look at them. Let's first realize that as we've opened other areas we've already prepared the neck and jaw for change. Do you remember occipital traction from an earlier releasing segment? Do you see how it's always appropriate?

Think of the hyoid muscles at the front of the neck: infra—sternohyoid, thyrohyoid, and omohyoid (we'll look at it specifically in the next chapter)—and supra: stylohyoid, geniohyoid, hyoglossus, and digastrics. Their names pretty well tell us where they're going. We seldom talk about hyoid muscles or bone, but it's sensible that they get shortened by a tight and forward head. If we can soften the hyoid muscle anywhere, we soften them everywhere. In the earlier diaphragmatic release we followed tissue up the back of the sternum to the sternohyoid muscle to lengthen the throat. And the last chapter's heart hinge turtle work is one more way we've worked toward this release. Now, work right at the chin and front of the neck is appropriate (Figure 11.1).

I've been working inside jaws for 25 years, and have found a protocol that makes sense for me. This chapter features late in the book because jaw release work isn't something I take lightly. It's life changing!

Here's another reason to open the throat: I suggest that keeping the heart out, head up, and throat open helps us release addictive behavior. Many of us try to numb a shortened deep line from head to waist with addictive behaviors to stifle our frustrations and cries for help. I'm remembering Mike, an angry and unhappy older alcoholic who worked with me to release his deep line so he could find and voice his anger. As he pulled his head out of his heart and freed his throat, he was finally able to express who he was and what he needed from his world.

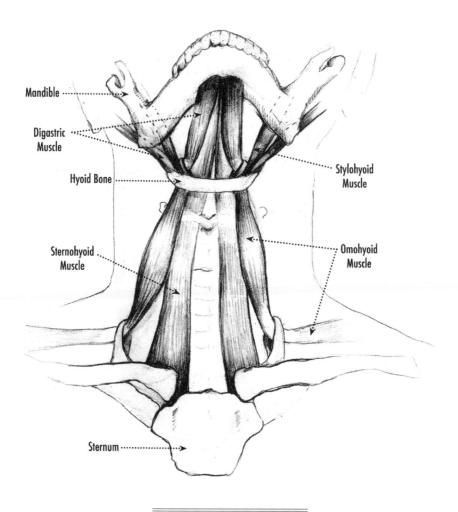

Mandible

Digastric
Muscle

Hyoid Bone

Stylohyoid
Muscle

Sternohyoid
Muscle

Omohyoid
Muscle

Sternum

### Figure 11.1 Front of the neck

*I sometimes see the infra- and suprahyoid muscles as the
psoas or spanners of the neck and throat. Can we create
length and resilience, or do we tighten them?*

## CORE fascial release of the jaw: Hold your tongue

1. Client is supine and gives permission; you're gloved and consistently remind them they're in charge. Teach them to stay open and relaxed at the deep line as you work. If they can't, don't work. Client staying reasonably relaxed is critical.

2. Explain each touch you make, what, and why. Remember, this work is far less about making large changes and far more about touching the client and teaching them to stay inside their body, breathing *while* you work in their jaw.

3. Insert index finger of one hand into client's same side jaw—R to R or L to L. Find pterygoids; visualize them forming an X and slowly, softly strum its center. Gently use corresponding finger of the other hand to coax the same line from outside the jaw. You'll affect masseter, buccinator, and zygomatic.

4. Come out for breath and rest. Then touch two: Trace with fingertips inside and behind the lower teeth. About halfway to the root of the tongue, you often find the "gag spot." Challenge it a bit, but let client win!

5. Side two both touches. Ask: Do you feel balanced? Still tight on one side? Can't tell? Use their feedback to see if you want to return to any spot with a slightly deeper intention. Mildly tug lower teeth up and forward (ceilingward) for three or four breaths.

6. Pull the hard palate up toward third eye for three or four breaths. I usually use my opposite hand to create traction on the occiput as I work this palate.

# ESCAPE

Addictions take us into a temporarily better place. They help us numb the past and future; the fear, boredom, anger, and shame. Addiction may not be totally bad if we're addicted to things that improve us. To what are you addicted? Is it helping to free you, or is it just keeping you from sharing your CORE with your environment?

While I don't believe it's a good idea to allow yourself to become addicted to *anything* that takes you totally out of yourself, it makes sense that some addictions have more positive potential than others. Yet an addiction to jogging when one has foot problems could be a tossup between positive and negative. I'm intrigued with the idea of evaluating an addiction to see where it fits on this constructive to destructive scale. Is it harmful or life-enhancing? And even if constructive, don't addictions and attachments still trap us in our core by numbing our bodies to the environment?

*Any* behavior can become addictive. The key questions to ask self are: Does this behavior take me further into or further away from myself and my truth? Is my addiction shielding my heart and CORE and creating false security? Is my relief and release long term or short term? Am I obsessed with maintaining a behavior? What will I do, or surrender, to maintain it? The answers to these questions give us good feedback about our addictions or attachments and where they're leading us.

## HOW BIG IS YOUR UNIVERSE?

I have a theory about "here" and "there." Mike had a small "here" (a tight core) and was mostly uninterested in a greater "there" (his larger environment). He grew up on a farm near a small town and never traveled far from home during most of his lifetime. He wasn't in the armed forces and never got used to staying overnight away from his own bed. To him, "there" was anyplace more than an hour's drive from home. He didn't really know much about that larger "there" world—he was content to live in the small "here" he knew well, and mainly saw "there" on television.

Many of us perceive a compact and safe "here" and see out "there" as dangerous and foreign. Evidently Mike's small "here" wasn't all he wanted it to be. Alcohol helped him travel, explore, express, and communicate between CORE and environment. I think if Mike had known a larger "there" naturally, he might have been happier in his life and less dependent on alcohol.

## WHAT WILL YOU EXPRESS?

What are your addictions/attachments? Even if you only admit to something mild, think carefully before you say "nothing." If you use a substance, behavior, or activity as a coping mechanism, perhaps you're addicted. Even meditation, altruism, or seeking self-esteem can be addicting. Make sure any behavior allows you to find and express yourself instead of numbing or escaping your core. I've long made a distinction between using a substance or behavior as a *sacrament* or an *addiction*. It's my goal to use *any* behavior or substance prayerfully to further know myself—the body and blood of Christ as a communion sacrament helps some contemplate Jesus' sacrifice. Using it mindfully makes it more special. The Native American use of peyote to take seekers into trances doesn't happen every evening! If someone uses their "sacrament" to expand "here" on a frequent time frame, they probably want to consider whether they're experiencing a sacrament, or are just addicted. I truly believe an addiction can be seen as a sacrament gone wrong.

Having a clear and honest head about what you're doing and how it's affecting you is important when you're serious about getting your here (core) to take up more there (environment). If behaviors help you escape yourself, an obvious question is, "*Why* do I need these behaviors in my life?" What pain or fear are you trying to numb or escape? It may be time to work on your mental as well as your physical tightening. Counselors, ministers, spouses, or friends: all can help you when you're ready to explore these concepts. Only after you've dealt with your own issues are you prepared to be present with love when similar issues appear in your clients.

## FIND THE CORE

Much of my work is based on the power of surrendering to *something* we can trust. If in the physical realm I endeavor to coax people to look at their painful spots, why wouldn't I want to do the same in the mental/spiritual/energetic realms? If we've gotten ourselves in a mess at the ego by tightening the head into the gut and pulling our throat into our heart, can we really trust the ego to get us out of this tightening? Shouldn't we lift our problems to a higher chakra's power to open and allow wisdom, expression, kindness, discernment, and creativity through us (keywords for chakras 6, 5, 4, 3, and 2)?

Surrender isn't easy, but it's necessary. For years my prayer group started each of our sessions with: "I surrender my will to the guidance of the Holy Spirit. My ego-self sometimes feels powerless and unable to solve perceived problems. I choose to have my ego-self step aside and focus my awareness on the Holy Spirit, my source of empowerment." Ask the client: "Do you feel how true surrender encourages the entire line to lift and open? Can you feel how, when safely connected to both the earth and to our higher power/crown/heaven, we unlock our gut, open our heart, and express ourselves to a greater world?"

Here are questions I've used to trigger serious surrender and release, both in myself and with clients:

- How do I get in my own way and waste my own energy?

- Do I create situations where I can denigrate or abuse myself or others?

- How do I self-sabotage? Who am I trying to please by maintaining this old behavior pattern? What old coping skills am I ready to discard?

- How much energy do I have in my: head, gut, heart, sex organs, arms? Do I starve an area? Why?

I'm sure you can think of other appropriate challenges to ask yourself, or clients, to release old habits. Specific words are less important than observing self (surrendering) and asking for guidance and honesty in dealing with the observations, so one can *admit to* (express) and *change* behaviors that aren't really serving one's Higher Good. "How have you stopped your own good from flowing through your bodymindcore? Put that question into your own words, and express your truth to free your throat from your heart, head, and gut."

Perhaps many of us hold on to addictions because we believe our energy should always be loving and joyous; we don't express whatever feels less than positive. Author Catherine Ponder, in her book *Open Your Mind to Prosperity* (1984), suggests one of life's greatest problems is congestion. She has a tremendous tool for helping us dissolve congestion and express resentment as we open our throat. She suggests we identify whom we feel has wounded us, and write a letter to the angel of this person. We don't confront the person or mail the letter. We simply write to their angel, expressing how we feel wronged and hurt by the behavior of their charge. After we've written the letter, we let it go! We don't go back and revisit—don't re-sent or re-send, yet don't re-scind.

Like Mike, many of us can't express anger, frustration, or resentment on our own. Hopefully you'll refer these trapped clients to a counselor or psychotherapist. Possibly they can just imagine their nemesis in an empty chair, and voice to that chair how they feel about the way they've been treated, and feel an acknowledgment of their pain. Maybe they can imagine a trusted adult from their past sitting with them to advocate for them. If we define our boundaries as to what's acceptable behavior from others, and really know and understand our bottom line, often those who've crossed that line in the past won't cross again. Somehow they sense the psychic bottom line we've expressed and they honor it. But first we must express it to our self!

Sometimes our throats need to express directly in a "heart to heart." In this case, it's usually productive to keep our messages in the "I feel" mode. Without attacking someone, we can tell them how we feel their behavior has affected us: "When you said that to me, I felt...(mad, sad, ashamed, guilty, stupid) because I needed...(support, validation, guidance). Was that your intention?" In this way our throat can express our core to speak for and unburden our heart.

Often when we ask for such clarification we'll immediately get a whole new perspective. Some people who've stepped on our toes did so unintentionally. If we express how we feel, they'll respect us and make a change in their behaviors. If they won't, we may want to rethink the relationship. If they treated us badly intentionally, we're in charge of setting boundaries that tell this person their behavior is no longer acceptable. We've trained others to treat us badly; we've now got to retrain them.

Realize too that sometimes the pendulum may swing a bit too far as we learn to set and express boundaries. We may make someone even more unpleasant toward us as we learn to assert ourselves and express our needs. We may occasionally err as we begin to be respectfully assertive. This isn't meant to stop us; it's meant to suggest we put ourselves in the other person's shoes and try to sense how we're being perceived. Are we demanding or petulant? Are we stubborn? Do we believe we can force someone to learn kindness? Good luck. Remember: "I felt…I needed…"

If we know our boundaries and respect the other person, and then learn to stay calm, focused, and on message, we'll have a better chance of being heard and responded to in a positive way. We can't assume we'll leave feeling satisfied with the other person's response. We only control our expression of ourselves. And as we learn to express clearly, we can more easily model clear expression for clients.

Say to clients: "Without judging self, discern whether you like who you've become…and if you're really brave, surrender and express these discernments to your higher self and to a friend. It's amazing how long a list might become when we look at ways we hold ourselves back. But relax and feel the feeling of open chakras throughout the body as you clear your throat to express and release."

- What congestions are you ready to clear out of your life?

- How are you wasting your own energy?

- How are you self-sabotaging, and who are you trying to please?

- Which coping mechanism is no longer serving you?

The throat chakra is one of the trickiest areas to work, partly because bodywork flirts with becoming psychotherapy when working with clients' expression issues. If you're present with love and encourage your clients (and yourself) to express honestly, you are serving their being...and your own. And remember: head upback and waist levelback while we uplift our hearts...only when these three centers (3/4/6) learn to stretch apart can energy flow between them as we "find our voice" and express our core. Let's continue to open and lengthen the central channel of our bodies so joy can flow through and out of us without our falsely creating it through addictive behaviors.

## Remember

- As we return to opening the head, gut, and heart centers and creating space and energy between them, we challenge our throat chakra to relax and express what we need and want.

- We allow our addictions and attachments because they help us numb our cores, cares, and dissatisfactions. A sacrament is meant to take us deeper inside *and* outside ourselves; overused, it becomes an addiction. Can you honestly discern?

- When you decide it's time to work on releasing that which keeps you from your greater good, an important first step is surrender: one of the most difficult decisions you may have to make.

- Look honestly at what's not working in your life: surrender and *express* to yourself and a friend.

## All purpose cue

"Look in a full-length mirror and ask for side-to-side balance in your body: make your hips look alike, your shoulders, your feet and knees. Cover one half of your face and observe; then cover the other side. Do you see two different people? Can you balance them? Look deeply into your own left eye in the mirror with only your left eye; then look into your right eye with only your right eye. Which side of you feels weak? Experiment with your right eye meeting your left eye in the mirror, and reverse. Ask your eyes to come forward, come out, meet you, and tell you you're all right as you are."

# Client challenge

### EASY

Begin to practice "expressing yourself" more; whether singing in the shower, talking to a pet, or standing up to whatever bully bothers you. Take small steps toward being heard.

### MEDIUM

Stand with your legs fairly wide apart (about 26–30 inches) and remain grounded in your inner leg line with the inner arches earthdown. Level yourself: pelvic bowl, waist, heart, and head. Allow the elbows to lead upbacklong and make a C curve that keeps the pelvis, gut, and heart frontout *while* feeling the stretch between the elbow/head and pelvis/inner arches. Now, sing or shout!

### DIFFICULT

Sit in a deck chair with arms. Allow your head to roll back in slow half circles while the canvas supports your back and shoulders. Eventually make a slow whole circle. Can you keep your low back back too?

### INTRIGUING

Allow yourself to discern parts of yourself you don't like. Perhaps you'll write them; perhaps you'll merely think about your current and past problems and behaviors. Before you share with a friend, stand before a mirror with your head up, waist back, and heart open to express your inventory with your own higher power.

### IMAGINE

What can you do for yourself, today, that challenges you to express yourself creatively?

CHAPTER
12

# SERVE WITH JOY

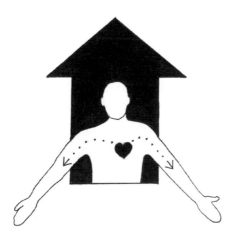

## WELL-OILED MACHINE—OFF, OR ON?

*Do we relate to our world in resentment, or in joyful satisfaction?*

*Holding onto resentment is like drinking poison and
expecting someone else to die. It won't work.*

Too many of us suffer from neck and shoulder problems. I've begun to believe they're one and the same—the neck problem anchored in the shoulders and the shoulder problem rooted in the neck; both tighten arms, hands, and even low backs. When we allow ourselves to work and express with open arms, in a relaxed flow, from the heart and throat, with a good head on our shoulders, we begin to release tension everywhere simply by doing what we love, with our heart, voice, back, and arms in it, in a relaxed process.

Years ago Mildred, an older client of mine, told me she didn't put any credence into Louise Hay's work, which I mentioned earlier. *You*

*Can Heal Your Life* (1984) has a glossary of physical conditions and diseases paired with an emotional origin or seed for the condition, and an affirmation one can use to dissolve that condition. Usually I feel Hay's observations are sound.

Mildred told me she didn't believe the book because "I have arthritis, which Louise Hay says is caused by resentment. Now, I'm not a resentful person. But if that *was* right, I could look around and see a lot of people who *should* have arthritis and don't." I didn't even try to point out to Mildred how her reasoning seemed like that of a resentful person, and to me she was proving Hay's point!

This chapter on arms speculates about what I call "Factor X"—the name I give to an unknown quality we each have or lack in varying degrees. The question I've asked myself is this: Why can some people survive 40 years working in a mine while smoking two packs of cigarettes a day and live to 90, while others shrivel and die from an upset stomach or an ingrown toenail? How do some resist the latest virus while others catch everything? What is that Factor X that lets some of us be healthy while others struggle, no matter how hard we try to take care of ourselves?

## LET IT GO!

To my thinking Factor X is, very simply, the ability to let SOAR energy flow through the entire bodymindcore. We all have the ability; Factor X is how well we can open the channel to allow that flow. Good energy flow manifests as good digestion and elimination, as freedom in the joints, as strong circulation, as healthy and happy thoughts and feelings in one's world, as a joyful and meaningful life. And it's tied to a large question: Do we relate to our world in resentment, or in joyful satisfaction?

Some people hold every thought and feeling, process every emotion to distraction, and stay in a resentful place. Some simply can't process and eliminate all the stimuli that come into their bodymindcore. Others are able to easily look at a situation, be it emotional or physical, take the proper nutrition from it *or* decide it's poisoning them, process and get the nutrition from the situation, dump out the waste product, and move on. Those who can do so have intuitively mastered Factor X on some level, and maintain better health. Those who get stuck in their process are dying more quickly. Put simply, we either live as if life thrills us, or scares us, to death.

Don't we hold on and hold on—whether to expectations for self or others, to old habits and survival skills we know aren't healthy, to ideas that no longer serve us, to relationships that take away our vital essence? The place we are feels comfortable, even when it's unsatisfactory, because it's known and within our rules. Embracing change sounds like it would take effort, so many of us do whatever we can to resist. My Factor X is an ability to roll with the punches, embrace the new, move through whatever stimulus comes our way, and be enthusiastic about the process. It's the belief that each experience is a piece of life to be tasted, evaluated, digested, and released.

In other words, Factor X is one's ability to replace fear and resentment with enthusiasm and gratitude. Factor X allows us to be engaged, not frightened. And for me, Factor X is best represented by the arms as they relate to the heart, and the way we serve with open arms or with a closed heart. Thus this chapter's logo person. Isn't it interesting that the Oriental Heart meridian ends at the fingers?

## REPLACING RESENTMENTS

Have you ever broken the word resentment into its components to better understand the meaning? Re-sent-ment is rooted in the Latin word "sentire" which means "to feel, experience, or hold an opinion." Add the prefix "re-" and you see resentment means feeling again and again. The suffix "-ment" means the state or condition. The definition as we've dissected the word therefore becomes: the state of feeling or holding again and again. And that's what resentment is and does—it makes you feel a feeling over and over. This definition doesn't have the negative connotation of the traditional definition, but I believe *any* time we feel again and again—positive emotions or negative—we're tying up our bodymindcores. That tying up of emotions is what we need to release if we want to add Factor X into our life equation.

To me there aren't "positive" and "negative" emotions or stressors. What's positive or negative is how "stuck" we get in any situation. I don't think it's healthy to be "stuck" in joy. I find people who seem to live in a world of forced enthusiasm to be less than genuine, and not always fun to be around. Likewise, those stuck in a negative world, even if genuine, aren't as easy to be with as they might be. The key is the word "stuck." How can we be authentic when we're stuck?

## BURDENS YOU SHOULDER: A PAIN IN THE NECK?

In a previous state of evolution I believe we humans were four-legged in relationship to our mother earth. From the time we've evolved from living on four legs until now, we've lost some ability in our front legs and their hips, the shoulders. This chapter will be longer because it contains a few extra stretches and awarenesses for shoulders and arms to make up for the loss of use too many of us bear today.

Think back to my earlier idea that one's arms can start as far down the back as the sacrum or tailbone, or as high up the body as the back of the head. This arm hinge seems to me a long and moveable hinge (Figure 12.1), encompassing all the chakras: When we reach for the sky we're reaching from the sacral/survival area. When we reach straight out, we reach with our hearts; when we reach down, we reach from our heads and throats. Every chakra governs and helps operate hands and arms, which move in different directions with various intentions. Keeping the arms open and free becomes vital to having a healthy back and core.

So arms reach from all chakras, especially the sixth (third eye), fourth (heart), and third (solar plexus): the three primary Chinese energy centers. When we put our shoulder into a job, we do well to come from the head, back, and heart. It's a much happier task and process when all the team's players are working toward the same goal; especially one they believe in. The brain allows us to decide what work to do and how much of it. The heart and thymus gland regulate the body's energy, and the stomach/back chakra regulates sweetness in one's work through the pancreas.

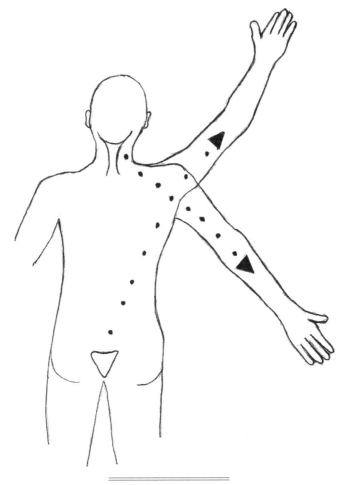

Figure 12.1 Arm hinge

*Remember, the arm hinge can initiate from many
points, depending on function.*

Arms, elbows, wrists, and fingers—all come from deep within our being. When we're not having fun with our work, we brace ourselves to the core. Which would you rather do with your body—"have your heart in your work," or "work your fingers to the bone"? The same work has a different toll on your body, depending on your attitude toward it. If we work in joy, relaxation, and gratitude, we massage *our* bodies with our works. If we work from frustration, resentment, or achievement mode, we create shoulder and neck pains, tennis elbow, carpal tunnel pain, arthritis, and spinal rotations as well as additional strain on the heart. All come from tightened and resentful arms.

## CORE fascial release of the arms: Reaching out

1.  Arm work can begin as low as the quadratus, latissimus, and erectors on the back and at obliques, rectus, and diaphragm on the front.

2.  Soften: Trapezius and pectoral muscles; then slower and more focused around serratus anterior, subclavius, and rotators.

3.  Now: Down one arm…beginning with deltoids, treat the tuberosity as an IT band of front leg. Soften it, realizing it too is very tender.

4.  Distal to elbow, find the interosseus membrane trough and work medial *and* down that line while client flexes/extends wrist.

5.  Find the thenar eminence, that spot between thumb and forefinger, and milk it toward yourself, pulling on a line to the heart, while client brings elbow slightly lateral and breathes. You may both feel a line all the way to the heart, if you allow yourself to try to find it.

6.  Second side.

7.  I will also work acromion processes or do jaw work to release arms.

## ELIMINATE NEGATIVITY

In Oriental medicine there's a point in the fleshy place just between thumb and forefinger called "the Great Eliminator." Squeezing and stimulating this point is said to relieve many congestions in the body, including headaches, stomach aches, and seasickness, cure hiccups, cleanse the liver, and even induce labor in a pregnant woman. I find it interesting that when I work with this point in clients I—and they—often feel a deep line of holding that travels through the arm and shoulder, all the way to the heart (Figure 12.2). Isn't it intriguing that the Chinese understood the need to "eliminate" negativity and replace it with positive energy thousands of years ago?

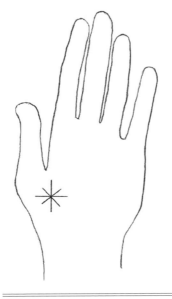

Figure 12.2 Great Eliminator point

*Learn to squeeze this point, move elbow slightly to the side, relax, and breathe to cleanse a deep arm line all the way to the heart.*

Find this spot for yourself. Simply squeeze the pad between thumb and first finger, just past the bones. Milk the tissue toward the fingertips—straight between the digits, next move along the side of the finger, then take a third trip down along the thumb. As you squeeze the pad, focus on opening your elbow slightly and trying to feel the line of holding that goes to your heart *while* you pull your head and neck longaway. Can you imagine at the same time you can "eliminate" negativity in your life and replace it with gratitude? And can you see how living in a state of non-stop achievement causes one to shrink and tighten the core, leaving less energy for the shoulders, arms, and hands?

A muscle that ties the arm and shoulder to the neck is the *omohyoid* (Figure 12.3), which originates on the last chapter's *hyoid bone*, in front of and just below the chin. It travels behind the *sternocleidomastoid*, then bends, dives under the collarbone, and anchors on the shoulder, under/behind the clavicle. This single muscle shows us how fully shoulders and neck are tied together, and how the head and neck are part of our arms. The omohyoid pulls the shoulders into the neck when the core is tight.

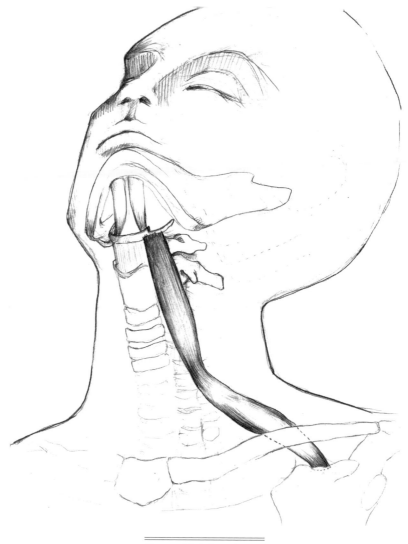

Figure 12.3 Omohyoid
*Can you see why neck and shoulder issues may be tied together?*

I've been dealing with quite a few frozen shoulders in clients recently, and have come to a conclusion that much that's "frozen" is fear of moving into and through pain. When I convince clients—and myself—to go fearlessly but respectfully into fearful places, we begin to unwind—arms, shoulders, neck, and heart.

## LESS MULTI-TASKING

Too many of us spend too much time trying to prove our importance and busy-ness to self and others. You can't walk down a street of a "civilized" city without nearly colliding with someone who's busily text messaging friends or checking emails on their Blackberry or iPhone. Several train accidents have lately been caused by engineers who were texting while driving. We've developed a habit and belief that single-mindedness is a waste of time. Not true!

We could learn to slow down, appreciate the task at hand, and bask in the satisfaction of each completion instead of looking at the overwhelming mental to-do list, and plowing ahead even harder. Often I say to a client, "You're an achiever, so this week, I'd like you to *achieve* relaxation. I'd like you to put on a CD, lie on the floor, listen to one full song while breathing, relaxing, and stilling the mind. You can't sort the mail, talk on the phone, make the grocery list, or do anything but relax. Do you think you can achieve that?" Occasionally I see the light go on, and know this person has finally heard someone tell them to slow down, let go of achievement mode, and enjoy their existence.

So how do we let go? How do we slow down and enjoy life? How do we dissolve resentment? How do we encourage clients to do likewise? First, we must realize and own that we've trained people, including ourselves, how to treat us based on that earlier factor: we're trying to duplicate what love or positive strokes looked like where we grew up. We're trying to recreate a pattern that may be damaging, but feels familiar. If Mom was abused by Dad, we may try to assume an appropriate role, becoming the abused or the abuser. If children should be seen and not heard, we may have chosen that model to raise our children. Too often, we recreate this fallacy of what love should look like.

If we allow ourselves to recognize we base current behaviors on long-ago patterns that are no longer the most effective way to operate, we can start to unwind these detrimental attachments and unresolved thought forms. If we'll remember to slow down to savor our tasks instead of worrying whether we're doing enough or doing well enough, we can breathe and relax. We can allow ourselves to soften the closed fists we created as we "dug in our heels" and "stood our ground"; we can decide to "put our heart into our work," and live a far different life.

## THE X FACTOR

British TV created the "X Factor," which has now come to the US. In it, judges and the public try to identify the most star-worthy performer. What is the X Factor? To me it's the star quality—do you want to look at this person, listen to them, and be around them? Do they exude energy and good feelings? Talent has a lot to do with success in the entertainment industry, but that X Factor is important too. We sense an authentic energy, or a lack of it, that makes us want to spend our time listening to and watching one person instead of flipping the channel. Star quality is based on this energy flow. Those who look successful and feel successful make us like them, because they have this X Factor.

And in a way the X Factor is that Factor X. Some people see the glass as half full; others see half empty. Some people see every aspect of their life as a bit of good fortune to be celebrated—even those parts that don't yet make sense. They exude joy, confidence, and optimism. They shine a bright light and sing a beautiful song. Others see trouble at every turn, so fears and resentments slow their energy because that Factor X ability to savor life has been trained out of them. They don't know how to allow energy, enthusiasm, and excitement for life to flow through their chakras, hinges, dantian, or core. We don't usually celebrate or admire these people.

## STRETCHING AT THE CORE

I add quite a few stretches in this chapter because I believe we work too hard with too little joy, and our shoulders and arms are burdened. Consider that we once used arms as front legs, and you see how the joints are still learning a new position. So, stretch in all ways! One profound way to stretch the arms from the core is to simply pull the shoulder blades skyup out of the seated/anchored sitting bones while maintaining equal weight in both hips. This seated stretch encourages spinal length and open chakras. We usually think our arms hang from our spine; can we stretch the arms and allow the spine to hang from them instead?

Another posture I like stretches many body hinges at once and coaxes all to release and relax (Figure 12.4). I stand and fold my arms over my chest; then begin to bend forward. I allow my elbows to fall away from my body earthlong to the floor as I work to stretch calves, knees, and hamstrings straightback, low and midback upback, head and neck downoutlong—pulling elbows floordown away from all. Work to feel hamstrings to toes first; next stretch hips and buttocks before finding and stretching back; finally shoulders. Let the elbows become a pendulum; front to back *and* side to side; then experiment with other penmanship patterns.

Simple rotating movements or shoulder rolls at the end of a long day, or session, or a long page or paragraph, can help me relax, breathe, and realize I've gotten stuck in achievement mode again. Think of Atlas, the mythical holder of the world, shrugging. I also see the benefit of using a broom handle, cane, umbrella, or any such "stick" at the back of your neck, with your hands holding the stick at its ends, behind your head. Swivel the stick, and your body (Figure 12.5). Twist in any direction you can find, breathing all the way…but invite the tension you've stored in the arms and shoulders to dissipate. Simple tools used with awareness can often replace sophisticated machinery.

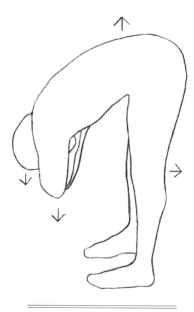

Figure 12.4 Bending stretch

*Don't try to touch your toes with this bend; get your hands out of the picture.*

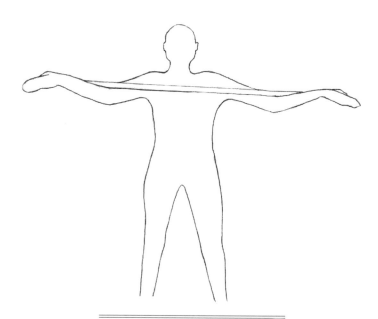

Figure 12.5 Stick behind shoulders

*Make this stretch up!*

Say to client: "Perhaps simplest of all, yet in some ways very complex, is the idea of resting one arm at the top or back of your couch, settee, or armchair, and stretching away from it (Figure 12.6). Allow its elbow to reach away from your spine, but vary the spinal segment from which you tug your elbow. In other words, pull your elbow sideways while you pull your head and neck the other way. Then bring your awareness a bit farther down your spine, to perhaps C7/T1, the 'dowager's hump' at the top of your shoulders. Pull any spinal segment in one direction *while* your elbow moves away. Experiment with using one finger or a thumb to lead: Move even farther down your spine to around your heart and again create space between elbow and spine. As you stretch from different segments, chances are you'll find one or two that really need this stretch. This is something you can do nearly anywhere, anytime."

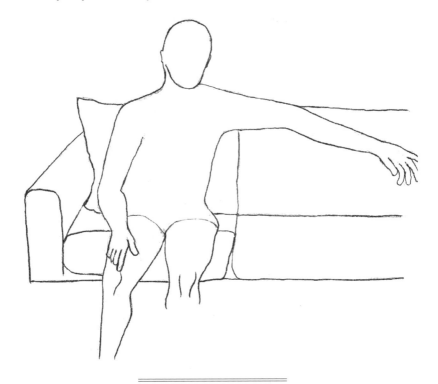

Figure 12.6 Arm over couch

*Place an arm on the couch, then stretch your head, neck, or back away from the arm.*

Lately I've also experimented with walking on all fours, and putting more weight into my front legs, or hands. In fact, as I pretend the fingers are toes, I find I don't know how to push off with my front toes and I'm heavy in the heels of my back legs. As I work to strengthen the fingers, and indeed the front legs, it seems I'm exercising muscles all the way up my arms and into the shoulders (Figure 12.7). Experiment for clients, and us: "Whether you're a long and flat animal, such as an alligator, or a tall and long-legged animal such as a giraffe, play with allowing more weight in the front legs *while* you hold the waist upback as you're walking. Don't neglect the back legs; shift weight from heels to toes, inside and outside arches, and from one leg to the other—in both front and back feet/hands."

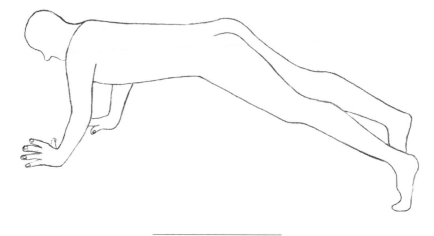

Figure 12.7 Animal walk

*The challenge is to keep the back straight and waist back; then pay attention to weight placement in the back and front feet.*

"And what if you next become a lizard whose front legs connect through the elbows? Can you crawl on and motivate only through your elbows? What if we'd evolved into a different creature that moved through and rested on elbows? Experiment with supporting yourself facedown on the floor. Now, raise toward the sky your head, shoulders, and spine *while* your elbows provide movement and support. Undulate: Experiment with moving spinal segments, including the head, back and forth/side to side *while* the elbows push down into the ground, the spine rises, and the tailbone pulls downlongaway from all." Connection: Could you do interesting shoulder/neck work with a client in this lizard position?

"To further your challenge, what happens if you sit on the floor, put your hands out behind you, and push yourself up into a bridge position with your belly uplong? Perhaps we could call this position a 'crab' (Figure 12.8). Can you feel how this reverse pushup stretches your shoulder girdles and challenges different muscles? Can you feel your shoulders responding? Can you also allow yourself to just 'hang around' in this posture and feel and observe the resistance in your shoulders? You can find a similar stretch by putting your hands on a table as you face away from it, and lifting."

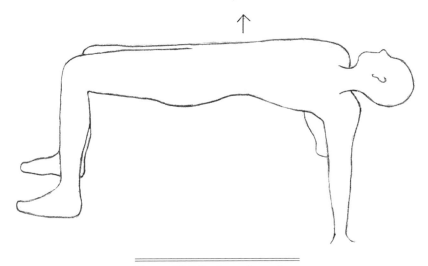

Figure 12.8 Backwards pushup
*A backwards pushup encourages a new set of shoulder muscles to waken.*

I've long been a fan of hanging from doorway frames or sturdier overhangs to stretch my shoulders, either together or individually, and allowing my spine to hang long at the same time (Figure 12.9). Lately I've also realized I can even hang from the shoulders, *while* I allow my spine to sag toward the floor, *and* lift my head uplong out of any of the spinal hinges that may be jammed (creating length between one and six). I even ask my head to make rotating motions that pull my third eye out of my own spine *while* I'm still asking the lower body to sink downlong into the floor. I've also begun pushing *up* into my fixed bar to positively stress my shoulders even more.

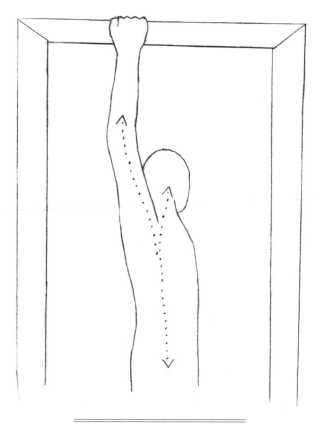

**Figure 12.9 Hang from doorway**

*Hanging from a doorway or bar allows the spine to hang off the shoulders instead of hanging the shoulders off the spine.*

Perhaps I'm getting lazier; perhaps wiser…but why not teach clients to practice stretching while sitting at a desk or table or deck chair, standing at a counter, or even sitting in an easy-to-move-into arm-chair? "Allow the elbows to rest on the surface, then lift your head and torso uplong off the elbows and feel the stretch up into the shoulders *while* the spine drops and hangs." If arms are front legs, many of us have lost the ability to let that front hip girdle carry us forward.

All these stretches can be effective, as can others in my client book *Meet Your Body* (2009), but the attitude you hold while doing them is most important to your health. Common sense tells us if Factor X is satisfaction with one's life and the ability to move through it happily, those who can't find satisfaction slow their own energy flow and become unhealthy more often than those who find joy in their activities. Factor X allows us to create communicative, loving relationships that make us feel supported, not resentful. I believe I've stumbled on a nearly perfect affirmation that you may have noticed already: "I'm satisfied with my progress and my process." Does this make sense? Are you thrilled to death, or scared to death? Does life make you want to sing, or scream? And the bottom line of back, head, shoulder, and arm pain can be simplified to this: "Learn to pull and hold the stuck pieces of your back up and back." So simple, so hard.

Consider that most of us hold one of four emotional postures when it comes to the shoulders: we either bring them downback (defiant), upback (fearful), downfront (weary), or upfront (timid or hurt). Few of us know how to allow our heads to fit and shoulders to hang straight down from a long head and neck.

So, if dis-ease is stagnant energy, are we going through life flowing from event to event, feeling to feeling; or do we stumble over every real or imagined roadblock, allowing our energy to slow and die? Do we resent, or are we grateful for all? Do we get excited by life and work to maintain an active role, or do we let life pass us by? I believe it's a life or death choice.

If my Factor X theory is true (and I try to live as if it is—sometimes successfully) it becomes our goal to learn to get excited about anything and everything that comes our way, then bring that enthusiasm and joy to our work, through our arms. We can turn loose of our familiar fear factor and replace it with Factor X—the ability to enjoy, relish, and celebrate every moment. We can find enthusiasm for each and every situation that comes to us. That Factor X not only draws health to us, but draws other healthy people as well.

Ask yourself, and challenge your clients: "Who am I hurting by holding onto my re-sent-ments—the negative feelings *or* the positive ones? Am I changing the person who's receiving my anger? Am I hurting them? Or am I just hurting me?" I think holding onto resentment is like drinking poison and expecting someone else to die. It won't work. And practicing gratitude is drinking the nectar of the gods. It could make us live a long time.

Do you see how we make our own choice? How do we serve? By finding service we want to reach for with the head, heart, gut, and groin! We serve by listening to our inner knowing, our heart's desire, and reaching out to those behaviors and people who make us feel vital and on purpose.

May we all learn to allow Factor X—that ability to embrace life without holding on too tightly or fearfully—to fill our bodymindcores in every moment. May we learn to be grateful for everything in our lives. May we be thrilled with our existence and our being in every breath. That's health. That's healing.

## Remember

- Since we've evolved from a four-legged existence into a two-legged one, we've asked our arms to take on new functions *while* losing some of their old abilities. Arms deserve our attention—from head to tail.

- "Re-sent-ment"—feeling a condition over and over again only makes us get stuck in unhappiness. There are no negative and positive emotions—only negative and positive responses. We can eliminate resentments from our life with Vitamin "G": Gratitude. Do we feed on Vitamin G or B negative?

- Factor X is the ability to be grateful, satisfied, and enthusiastic with one's life. Factor X draws to us more to be grateful for and enjoy.

- Any stretching of the arms, hands, elbows, or shoulders that encourages the release of the head, neck, heart, and even groin can help you to clean your core/chakras/dantian/hinges and be ready to approach your work more enthusiastically.

# All purpose cue

"Find a stretching routine that asks you to use arms and shoulders in ways you don't normally move. Whether hanging from a desk or doorway, pushing your body up into a backward bridge, or simply using shoulder rolls, pay attention to your arms. Remember: working to *push* with your arm muscles stretches them too."

# Client challenge

### EASY

Look honestly at your work and your life. Are you enjoying them? If the answer is no, do your head, neck, shoulders, and/or arms hurt you? There may well be a correlation between your pain level and your joy level.

### MEDIUM

Experiment with sitting in a desk chair (though any posture will work). Pull your little finger's nail longaway from your elbow. Now tug the elbow outlong to the side as you still pull on the finger and try to feel a stretch all the way to the shoulders and ears *while* you move the opposite ear upaway, and breathe. Move your head around; make the tug from the finger and elbow consistent, yet experiment with realizing your deep arm line's tension.

### DIFFICULT

Stand with your legs apart and hands reaching skyup. Wrap one hand's fingers around the other wrist and let that wrist and hand reach upoutside. While stretching these fingers out of the shoulder, draw a circle upoutside with this hand.

### INTRIGUING

Practice catching yourself in any task or posture, seeing if you're balanced or putting all your energy into one side. Experiment with carrying your coffee cup down a flight of stairs in the "wrong" hand, or crossing the "wrong" leg, or holding the phone to the "wrong" ear. How does it feel?

## IMAGINE

I believe many of us use our right arm to achieve, to strike out, and be our offensive tool. Conversely, many of us use the left arm not only to receive, but also to shield ourselves, to cover our eyes, to defend. What would happen if you tried to reverse this position and ended up allowing the left arm to be the aggressor and the right to be the defender? Does it feel strange to you to reach or strike out with the left hand? Perhaps it's time to examine the roles we make our bodies play.

CHAPTER
13

# SO NOW RELAX

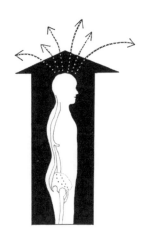

## JUST BE YOU—SURVIVE, OR THRIVE?

*Chemical changes in the body and brain are
triggered by attitudes as well as functions.*

*The more we remove kinks and clutter from our
body's core line, absorb shocks, and convert them to
information, the more freely all energies can flow.*

Now we come to my hero, chakra 7: crown. Whichever type of
authority one sees as most effective—God, general, governor, guru—
this highest chakra represents that wisest and most seasoned ruler of
the body community. I equate crown chakra health to the entire being's
overall wellness. When we find and operate from our crown, when we
"rise above" our problems and fears, we can truly learn to relax and live
in the present moment, free of the past.

I've mentioned CORE Energetics and the Center Of Right Energy, and my sense of humans as three-layered beings: core, body, and environment, with the body mediating between core and environment. We have sickness and pain in our bodies because they're tired of protecting our wounded cores from our uncertain environment. I've suggested psychological stretching, but have tried to ground that work in physical tissues.

Jim Oschmann, an early mentor, traces the science and history of the healing use(s) of energy in his book *Energy Medicine: The Scientific Basis* (2000). In regards to the connective tissue or fascia of the body with which I work, he says: "The more flexible and balanced the network (the better the tensional integrity) the more readily it absorbs shocks, and converts them to information rather than damage" (p.64). In other words, a balanced system contributes to our ability to convert trauma into information to be processed and eliminated instead of stored and feared. If this statement is true for the fascial system or network, isn't it also true for other systems including chakras and emotions?

Our crown was mentioned in an earlier chapter featuring chakra 6, the third eye, which rationally guides the body (hopefully in communication with number seven's higher power). Move above the head to seven, associated with the brain, cranial nerves, and *pineal* gland, which functions as a primary governor for the body as it regulates waking and sleeping functions, seasonal disorders, and light sensitivity. The crown also hopefully communicates with the root or survival chakra: while "Are we surviving?" from chakra 1 is balanced by chakra 6's "Are we thinking rationally?" above them both is the crown's "(We/I) consciously thrive without limits." Limits are what we allow others to set on us. Can we find our balance between pride and humility as we operate from our crown?

I see the root and sacral chakras as the negative junction box of our body's spinal column and the head as the positive junction. Thus our spine forms an electrical/energetic circuit. We can label this circuitry as meridians, nadis, channels, chakras, or core. We can touch a bone, muscle, blood vessel, nerve, or core. Whether none or all of these hold the elusive SOAR energy, therapeutically it makes sense to challenge the deep line respectfully when appropriate to continue to release stagnation through all networks. The more we remove kinks and clutter from our body's core line, absorb shocks, and convert them to information, the more freely all energies can flow. With an open crown we feel enlightened and connected to both heaven and earth. With a clogged crown we're separated from Oriental medicine's head, heart, gut, and groin, as well as chakras at the base and throat.

Do you see how well this idea correlates with classical Oriental medicine, where all the meridians which incorporate organs flow either up or down the body? Did you realize all these meridians are incorporated into one grand continuous circuit that travels up and down the body many times as it delivers energy?

Had you considered most kings wear a pointed crown that seems to invite energy from a higher power? Do you recall that bishops and other church officials often wear a mitre or headgear that seems to elevate their height, but also draw them nearer to heaven? Even witches wear pointed hats to invoke this higher power! Is it possible other cultures with tall headdresses may be attempting to expand crown chakra awareness? Many of us are skeptical of creating or maintaining a relationship with a "higher power"—we don't quite trust someone or something somewhere above us to manage our affairs, so give power to our lower centers instead. Yet in many ancient testaments, a hero goes to a mountain or higher place to make important decisions… isn't he also seeking to get above his problem and operate from this higher chakra?

While in Oriental medicine the heart is the Emperor, in my model the crowning chakra is indeed the "higher power" from which we could rule our energetic being, instead of from that physical emperor, the heart. If you're uncomfortable with God, or a higher power, imagine that the highest power in you is trying for the good—stay out of its way, and let its ideal be your ideal in and through you.

## LET THE CROWN RULE

If the message of this book can primarily be summarized as "Pay attention to and keep moving energy through the physical and emotional bodymindcore," the message of this chapter is specifically: "Teach clients to rise above the energetic clutter of their past and present bodymindcore restrictions to let the crown rule the entire core." One task serves the other. When we truly pay attention to our bodies, we realize *we* stop the flow of energy through our core line in much the same way we stop the flow of energy through our mind.

When trauma threatens us, a warning signal may present itself. We may truly be in danger, but perhaps our system is wound too tightly based on past experience, forcing us to overreact to *any* challenge. First our body releases chemicals that help us fight the perceived danger by increasing our blood pressure. Second in this fight or flight response of the adrenal system is to shorten breath; next we tighten the core as we assess and decide to stand or run. Too often we dig in the heels to stand our ground and fight for survival—if not physically, at least emotionally or energetically. If every step in our life seems like danger (and for too many of us, it does seem this way), we're living in survival (achievement) mode, not relaxed flow. But a wise ruler rarely loses his head over perceived threats, and that's why he's in charge of the community: the body.

Say to clients: "Consider allowing *your* crown to be your personal higher power and manage your life. I've already suggested you could see yourself as either the general or the foot soldier, sticking your neck out to get your head blown off, or watching from above in safety. Which do you want to be? Who rules you: merely surviving, or easily thriving?"

## ANOTHER TWIST OF THE MIND

I'd like to open another discussion about mental health here. It's yet one more way we get our heads turned around and choose surviving over thriving. Like toxic unresolved thought energies that come from the outer world, this condition—Alzheimer's disease—speaks to me of a thought process gone awry, from within.

What's Alzheimer's about anyway? My metaphor for this disease, this slowdown of mental energy, is filing cabinets. Some of us are afraid to throw away anything, including memories. We stuff each mental scrap into a file. After a long and full life, it can get difficult to retrieve the relevant scraps. Where did I file that memory? Which drawer? Which room? Some Alzheimer's sufferers can tell you clearly all about their childhood, describing in detail their fifth birthday party, yet can't recognize their children. Or they see their grandchildren and think these are their children, not realizing they've lost several rooms full of filing cabinets that covered years of their lives. Sometimes they can still navigate the early filing system before too many memories overwhelm it; eventually there are simply too many unprocessed information bits in their system. While an overstuffed filing system is probably not a conscious choice, nevertheless I believe many of us are overwhelmed by rooms full of stored irrelevant data and so can't stay in the moment because, at some point, we gave up on staying current in sorting data.

Have you ever considered that animals perform a function, then leave it in the past? Humans, on the other hand, recycle the tape of a function to see if they could have performed more diligently, happily, fully. This loop of worry creates the opportunity for trapped energy. Perhaps we've forgotten how to find neutral in our bodymindcores.

## PAY ATTENTION!

*Why* do we clutter our minds? Let's visit the "Nun Study" documented in the book *Aging with Grace: What the Nun Study Teaches Us about Leading Longer, Healthier, More Meaningful Lives* (Snowdon 2001), which follows a group of nuns who lived together and were observed for many years. Since they'd been in a controlled setting, they made a great study group—diet, schedule, hours of sleep, purpose; many factors were similar for the whole group. The results are thought-provoking.

Research showed that when these nuns died and were autopsied, some had the disease of Alzheimer's in their tissue but exhibited no symptoms; no memory loss or inability to function in the world. Yet others with milder cases of the disease, according to autopsies, weren't functioning mentally. What was the hidden factor? Research showed it was their intention to be involved in their current worlds.

In other words, those who made an effort to keep up with the world were less likely to be left behind and were current in the world. Those interested in the world around them and wanting to expand it died with disease in their tissues but not in their minds. Those who continually sought a smaller world or were overwhelmed by the larger one seemed to have shrunk further and further into earlier file rooms in their bodyminds, and lost the ability to keep up with later relevant memories and ideas. Those able to manage only a small "here" and shut off the world out "there" suffered a mental shrinkage, reinforcing the claim that chemical changes in the body and brain are triggered by attitudes as well as function.

Alzheimer's is yet another congestion. Like lack of communication in a relationship, a heart that wears out from unhealthy foods and too little exercise, a gut that's tied in knots due to bad chemical or emotional nutrition, or a mind that's either racing in its desire to prove its worth or has given up: A cluttered and overstuffed body, mind, or bodymindcore may congest, slow down, and decay. When we retreat deep inside ourselves instead of accepting, sorting, and releasing all the energy that swirls through us, we begin to die. Sometimes our mind CORE wears out before our body CORE, from lack of organization and/or stimulation—from lack of crown energy.

Perhaps those with Alzheimer's have lost the ability to reach their crown, so operate instinctively from a lower chakra: often survival, sex, or gut. Their seventh or crown chakra is overwhelmed by their brain and third eye, tightening the entire system and depriving the brain of energy. Maybe they simply can't stimulate themselves to find their higher power chakras anymore or release the unresolved thought forms they've allowed to settle into them. Possibly due to an atlas wedge at the sixth chakra (Chapter 6) they've congested their system, and the elevator is jammed just below the penthouse!

## BEAUTY, ORDER, HARMONY

Congestion comes in many forms. We all know packrats who can't seem to throw anything away. They surround themselves with things too numerous to sort, and never let any of them go, no matter how useless they might really be. How can one relax in such a situation and setting?

Others create "beauty, order, and harmony" in their world. They feel it's important to have surroundings reflect these values and choose items, people, and situations that contribute a higher vibration to the beauty, order, and harmony of their universe.

Which do you want to be? Do you absorb your work and home space and feel calm, or do you enter them and feel jangled? I love to look up from my work at the room or objects in it and feel a flood of peace, joy, and gratitude in my soul. The external environment becomes a mirror to the internal CORE universe we've created. Chaos outside? Chaos inside. And how does the body deal with that chaos? It becomes a barrier; body and core energy will descend toward survival when there's too much chaos in the environment. Chaos anywhere contributes to chaos everywhere.

In order to enhance our mental health, can we learn to mindfully keep only truly useful things and thoughts, and let the used-up or unused go on to their greater good; be that therapist, trashcan, charity shop, or a friend who will use it? Do kings really hold onto old clothes or broken furniture? Let go of that which isn't truly serving you, be it stuck emotions, junk, relationships, weight, or static energy of any kind: Move it! Allow yourself to get interested daily in the new world around you instead of constantly trying to preserve your old one. Create new energy that's incompatible to the old way of being.

I've thought lately we could all create a personal weekly "backflow day." Some of us do this on Sundays by attending church to tend our spiritual needs and seek reconnection. Perhaps we simply need a sunday where we go out and play in the beauty of nature. Church-goer or not, could it be possible to take one day a week to pay attention to what you've taken in during the week, physically and emotionally, and work with intention to process and eliminate all that's come into you? The Western style of living, particularly, encourages the collection of clutter in our lives—mind, body, and surroundings. Can we take the time on a regular basis to sort this collection and streamline our lives? Can we give clients the same challenge?

Can we learn to forgive our mistakes and wrong choices, and ask our higher selves more often and more quickly, "Where does this action, thought, or feeling register on my 'Feed My Soul' meter? Is this enhancing my life or slowing my energy? Am I relaxing or tensing because of this thought or feeling? Do I want to continue with this behavior or eliminate it? Is it helping me thrive, or merely survive?"

## EMBRACING THE SHADOWS

Carl Jung added the term "shadow" to the therapeutic vocabulary. I understand the shadow as those parts of our personality we've rejected, masked, or buried because of our own fears, ignorance, shame, or other lack of love moving through us. If we made a list of all the parts of ourselves we didn't like and worked to find the gifts and positive sides of these shadow parts, we'd integrate into our bodymindcore in yet another way. If we didn't possess a quality, we wouldn't see it in another; and what we see in another is a reflection of what we see—or are afraid to look at—in ourselves.

A tool to lighten the shadow experience might be to list all the reasons we can't do or be that which we'd like. Only after we sort and pare our inner objections, fears, and barriers, and allow them to speak to us, can we clearly see our path ahead. When we discard our resistances, amazing things can happen in our world.

Challenge clients to make those lists and ask their higher center: "What are the things you really want to do with your life? What are the obstacles and objections? Where are the shadows?" Encourage them to write them down, honestly. Do they want to continue these old beliefs, or are they ready to throw light on their shadows and change? Is it time to clean the physical and mental files?

## INTEGRATION

Integration is such a fascinating word to me. It implies we're bringing all the parts together in a new, more efficient way. At this stage of the book, that's exactly what we're trying to do—to ask the crown to stay in communication with the rest of the body, and to help all chakras/centers remember to relax and work together in a more efficient and harmonious style.

Let's not forget the related word "integrity." While we normally consider integrity to be related to honesty and truthfulness, do you see how it can be seen as a large component of integration? When we're living with our body relaxed and communicating with both itself and the bodymindcores outside our own, we're also living in integrity.

Physically, when we bring integrity to a body, a challenge often arises. Most massage therapists, and many other therapists, have gotten trapped by the acute problem client, the one who asks us to work on the problem spot for the entire session. At the end of that session, the problem may or may not be better, but we become aware that we've ignored much of the body's overall needs in our desire to "fix" their spot. Let's keep in mind that integration suggests we want to give attention to every part of the body (or psyche) in each session, whether we touch it or not. If we've worked left, we must work right (feminine/masculine); if upper, touch the lower (thrive/survive). If we've worked back at length, we must remember the front (physical/emotional). And if we've worked deeply, we must integrate superficially before we send the client back to their world (core/environment).

So, keep in mind that we're ready to see clients in a new light, asking them to examine the issues we find in their bodymindcores and decide what they want to do with them. Can we continue to challenge our clients to make changes in their world without tearing it apart? Can we coax them to integrity as we attempt to help them integrate their bodymindcores to make them healthier, happier, more free individuals?

My Universe truly is this simple, as I ask self and clients: Energy either moves through or slows down; where is yours? Where do you want it to be? How can you make changes? When will you begin? Stand on the hill and watch the drama unfold without losing your head. Stay above, but be aware of it all.

## Remember

- We tend to congest our lives and worlds in our need to hold onto thoughts, feelings, people, possessions, and attitudes. As we relax, sort, digest, eliminate, and reintegrate, we create health.

- We may accept Alzheimer's disease in our bodymindcores because we can't keep our mental and emotional files tidy.

When we surround ourselves with beauty, order, and harmony, it's easier to remain joyfully in the present moment.

- See the crown or guide chakra as the top of your electrical circuit and the root and sacral chakras as the bottom. Is your energy flowing freely between the two ends, or is it stuck? Can you let the highest chakra (thrive) rule instead of the lower ones (survive)?

- Embrace your shadows. Make lists of the aspects of yourself you don't like; ask why they're still happening, and what you can do to change them. And remember to *play* with releasing them, as you adjust your mental attitudes.

## All purpose cue

"I'd like you to consider this question again: What part of your body arrives first? Some few of us lead with our hearts; more lead with their heads and hide their hearts. Too many people lead with the gut, others the groin or even the feet. Which part leads you, and has it changed since you've been working with this book? Conversely, where does your fear live, and where do you hide? When you find answers for yourself, change something. Try a new way of being. And remember to relax and play with it."

## Client challenge

### Easy

Allow yourself to do some ruthless sorting in one area of your life, large or small: a thorough cleaning of a cupboard, drawer, closet, or garage. You may be ready to change an old relationship or practice forgiveness. Perhaps you simply want to clean your car, or one room, so you have one beautiful, orderly, and harmonious space.

### Medium

Take up that space. Sit or lie down, making sure you have plenty of stretching space around you. Think of your body as being comprised of two triangles: arms/shoulders to tail is one triangle and head to hips/heels is the second. Can you begin by lengthening either triangle? Pull your low back/tailbone downlong *while* you pull your arms upover. Pull your heels downlong *while* you pull your head upback. Experiment with pulling various points from your center.

### DIFFICULT

Stand on balanced feet; then level the pelvic bowl, waist, diaphragm, and head—level and skyup all chakras at once.

### INTRIGUING

Have you yet come to a feeling or belief that you're good enough and do enough?

### IMAGINE

See yourself as the ruler of your Universe, operating from and living in the crown. A ruler rarely worries about safety; he or she knows he or she will be protected.

# CHAPTER 14

# WHAT WE'RE HUNGRY FOR...

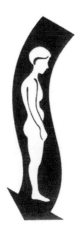
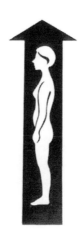

## MOVING FORWARD

*You'll never be fully healthy if you allow your past to keep you from living responsibly and joyfully in your present.*

*Cell by cell, we encourage the opening of that mid-body diaphragm to facilitate communication between segments.*

I'd like to close with a few words to tie our personal bodymindcore, therapist worlds into our larger world community, and to further challenge you to work on yourself in your own body instead of working on yourself through your clients' bodies and minds. I believe we're all cells in a universal tissue which some models would call a hologram of the larger whole or a microcosm of the macrocosm. In the chakra model we could consider the idea that we as a species are moving from lower chakra living through to higher ones, then out into our crown and our overall aura. Whichever model we use, it makes sense to ask each individual cell to operate for the good of the whole.

An old Chinese curse is reputed to be "May you live in interesting times." We've arrived there, haven't we? The world's financial system is melting down; the planet is being poisoned, and rebelling; politics is becoming more polarized; religions are demanding fundamental adherence to their tenets; and millions of children are being deprived of their opportunity to grow and thrive. We've lost our personal energetic connection to natural energies. No wonder so many of us are sick and tired: fearful, shamed, angry, jealous, gluttonous, greedy, and/or prideful. I'm reminded of another Chinese word with a dual meaning: crisis/opportunity. We're there too.

Consider overlaying the chakra system on our human species instead of on us as individual cells of that species. Currently upper and lower chakras don't seem to want to communicate with their opposite: the lower, survival chakras seem separated by an hourglass or diaphragm from the upper, thriving chakras so the two groups can't work together. Yet one must have a personal connection and communication between chakras 1–6 to be able to operate at seventh and eighth chakra awareness. All need to operate from a higher place *and communicate!*

*Neither* group seems to consistently find the crown chakra area which serves the good of the whole. Too many of us seem to be stuck in a specific chakra/center and tension/belief system. It's time for all the chakras to become integrated and coexist. If we're unwilling to change our opinions and move from our comfort zone or comfort chakra, can we give others the same courtesy without slamming the gate between belief systems? The most helpful gift we give others is to allow them to be who they are. Disagreement shouldn't stop us from listening and seeking areas of agreement.

It's my hope that society is beginning to open the hourglass between the lower, survival chakras and the upper, thriving ones. We're learning to allow that chakra elevator to stop at all the floors, yet be ruled by the highest power instead of whichever of the six lower centers we've tended to be stuck in and operating from. While many of us want to resist the idea of living in the entire bodymindcore and prefer our small universe based on whichever chakra center feels "safe" to us, I remind us again: Pain is resistance to change. If we're stuck in survival mode, it's time to learn to thrive. If we're stuck trying to bring others into thriving, it's time to look at our survival issues. And all can be served by learning to operate from that higher consciousness or power, the crown center.

As therapists, I believe it's essential we help our clients find and open their CORE essence spot at the diaphragm so they communicate between the upper body and lower; then activate the heart communication between self and environment (others). This is the healing work I believe we're invited to do: Cell by cell, we encourage the opening of that mid-body diaphragm to facilitate communication between segments and ideologies. It's time to heal!

The eighth major chakra is the overall body's *aura*. It's the part of each of us that resonates through the body with the greater world—our environment. While we've become relentless in the pursuit of the enhancement of *me*, I feel we'd all benefit if we'd gently work to pursue the enhancement of *us* and keep our eye on the whole game, not just our little area. For too many of us, *me* is more important than *us*. Current political debates show too many of us can't work toward a bottom-line goal we all agree on, because we're afraid of losing our personal piece of the pie in negotiations along the way.

Can we learn to recognize a common far-away goal and work backwards from that goal to negotiate through our differences or blocks (expansion of environment/large there) instead of operating from a fearful space (tight core/small here) that demands our viewpoint and goal is honored first and foremost (short and tight)? Why can't we learn to respect that every viewpoint, like every chakra, is worthwhile and has something to teach us all, yet none has all the answers? That the more we dialog, negotiate, and integrate, the more we're all enhanced? Why can't we listen to and honor every part of our own bodymindcore so we can respect and encourage the CORE of others? Why can't we mix our vital energy with that of others without fearing we'll lose ourselves? And, to be truly ethical, can we admit that too often we cause our own dilemmas? In Oriental medicine, health depends on sending positive chi energy to everyone, all the time.

As you've stayed with me this long, you know my belief in attitude is a large part of my philosophy. That which we focus on expands: If we focus on weariness and selfishness, we'll find more of it. If we're selfless and clear-hearted, we're healthy; if we're angry and judgmental, we're not. If we focus on the joy and abundance of our lives, more will be added. And if we can truly believe we deserve joy and operate from this belief, life is magnificent. Most of us have survived stressful periods. How can we trust more quickly that we'll survive, and thrive in satisfaction? How do we find rest, relaxation, and peace more often?

Psychologist Alfred Adler used to tell depressed patients that he could cure them in two weeks if they'd spend their time trying to make others happy. He suggested people who can't care about others are hurting themselves, but also hurting us all.

Many of us on the planet live from a place of depletion—we're so overworked, overstressed, and overextended that we often resent any request for help. "How can others demand of me? I've got nothing left to give." I understand we need to fill our own cup to overflowing first so we can nurture others from overflow instead of lack. How do we create, and keep creating, that overflow? How can we feel good about serving others when we need service ourselves?

It's time to learn to focus on enhancing "us" instead of "me." It's time to remember our individual cell is part of a larger tissue and organism that we best serve by nurturing the greater good instead of our individual needs. It's time to add service to others, or at least tolerance and respect for them, to our purpose. When we live in gratitude, won't we express generosity?

Challenge yourself to accept that you may not get it right the first time, or even the second. But if you stay on task, stay positive, and stay in community, you enhance yourself and us all. Staying in community requires us to communicate with and respect all others; to listen with two ears twice as much as we speak with one mouth. We can communicate and negotiate positively instead of negatively: to listen, process, and *compromise* so *all feel validated* instead of fighting for our personal agenda all the time. This is true integration, and also good therapeutic technique.

It seems some world leaders are beginning to understand these concepts. While they probably won't change the world quickly, I hope they challenge us to consider how the void in ourselves could be filled by respecting others, and the gifts we'd receive by so doing. Succeed or fail, they challenge us all, as I'm challenging us now, to begin to live life as if we're living first for the good of the entire human race, above our own bodymindcore self-interests. All can feather their own nest; but realize we can carry out this feathering in a win/win mode so we're not stealing feathers from someone else. For too long now, people higher in the power pecking order have had no consideration for those lower than them. It's time for reorganization from us all.

## A WORLD CHALLENGE

In the United States, I don't perceive we've had a unifying national challenge since the Second World War. This was the last time our nation came together as a common family for a sustained period of time, to rise above personal differences and labor for a common good and common goal. Roles were stretched: women became factory workers; men and boys manned the trenches and flew planes; children collected metal scraps; old people gardened, sewed, and raised grandchildren; all had a purpose, a task, a contribution to be made. Only once since the Second World War, on September 11, 2001, has the US citizenship been so united. Unfortunately, we didn't know how, as a people, to turn that tragedy into the next great undertaking for the collective body known as the US. What an opportunity was lost!

Now, simultaneously, I perceive four large and intertwined objectives for all of us; not just for the US. First, I believe we must soothe the sixth or mental chakra financial crisis (greed/charity) that threatens to bring us all down, by retooling and learning to be satisfied living within our means instead of coveting more.

Second, I believe what has been termed the "war on terror" (first or survival chakra: fear/diligence) must be reframed into a necessary dialog where we all commit to resolve conflict, whether that be through negotiation or last-resort fighting. This "war," as I see it, is about others' need to force us to be the people they want us to be, and our need to force them to be like us. We can't give them our individuality; we can't demand theirs from them either. We must somehow learn to coexist respectfully.

Third, I believe many in the world understand the fifth chakra, throat-level creativity crisis/addiction to consumption in our environment (gluttony/temperance), so are making calls to retool and create an environmentally saner footing. Again, our problems have come from our need to consume ever more hungrily to fill the internal emptiness that external expressions can assuage but never satisfy.

Fourth, I think change will come when we challenge ourselves to heart chakra service to others (envy/kindness), and by doing so, challenge each other to become better, more tolerant world citizens in community. If we can learn to remember how to serve that which is bigger than us, and to be more satisfied as we consume less, we're all enhanced.

## DUTY TAKES A RAP

Various groups understand this challenge to serve—religious organizations often "call" members. Political parties make a great display of rallying the faithful. Armed service for country is another greater-than-self calling. Ethnic and civil wars, though not fulfilling the requirements of service to the greater good, certainly call for service to their community, their organ. But too few individuals or societies have served the world's good in recent years. It's time to sacrifice a bit of *me* on our way back to service to the *us* whole.

Duty and sacrifice aren't words many people respond to positively. Take a few seconds right now to stop, think about the words, look away from the book, and notice your feelings as you think of them. Did you have a positive or a negative experience around them? Too often these words invoke an image of "must-do" as opposed to what makes our souls sing. Why can't we learn to believe duty and sacrifice can also make our souls sing?

I challenge you—and me—and clients—to live purposefully, in service to others, to the planet, and to the greater good. Since I believe it's preferable to be peaceful and happy within yourself before you serve others, I challenge you to be happy within yourself. Whatever has held you back from your own happiness, I say, "Get over it. Get on with it." You'll never be fully healthy if you allow your past to keep you from living responsibly and joyfully in your present.

I know this has a harsh sound, but I believe in the importance of living in the present instead of the future or past. In our present, too much of our pain is anchored in the past or future. *We can let it go.* Whether you feel you have a positive past or a negative one, I challenge you, and me, and clients, to live responsibly and fully in a positive present. As you release past behaviors, hopefully you'll discard held attitudes which kept you rigid in your thinking; as you allow others to have their opinions and feelings without making them wrong, you soften your own bodymindcore as you respect and contribute to your environment instead of fearing it. And as you clear your past behaviors and patterns, you're far better equipped to help others as they try to clear their own.

And remember, one of the best ways to take your mind off your pain or your negative here-and-now is to try to assuage the pain of others, to serve. If you didn't believe this at some level, you wouldn't have chosen the path of a therapist. Let's remember we can help others and work together to create the world we want to share. Let's remember to feel grateful so we can be generous.

## PRACTICING INDEPENDENCE WITH INTERDEPENDENCE

I return to the image that we're all cells in the planet body. Our specific tissue may be our family, our state, our community, our work group. The entity is greater than the cell. The cell must be healthy and productive, but in service to the nutrition of the tissue, and ultimately the whole. Too often we forget we're only one small cell of something greater. Let's remember we all share the planet, the times, and the determination of what our time on the planet brings us. Let's remember satisfaction, gratitude, and service as worthy attributes to develop and refine inside our own cell. Let's learn to keep our personal cell healthy and whole so the larger being can also be nurtured and thrive, as we learn to work in cooperation to achieve greater heights in the entire organism.

It's been my intention in this book to challenge you to think about developing, in self, then in clients, healthy survival skills—changing what served previously, but may no longer be appropriate. I've offered tools to help you and clients let go at physical and emotional levels; to restore the pure essence or CORE of your soul, to realize your worth, and to understand your contribution to the entire organism. Believe: You owe it to us to become the best "you" you can become. Each of us does. Anything less is not only self-defeating, but diminishes us all. Enhance us all—be yourself fully. To me, this call defines redemption. We don't have to shout about redemption to others when we feel worthy of it. We're all reaching for a common goal.

I have no reason to compete with you for the Universe's blessings, and I believe you have no reason to compete with me. I can like myself just as much as you like yourself. The Universe has enough to give us all what we want, if we honestly ask, strive to stay open to its good, and make a commitment to live in the present, fearlessly. May it be so.

Be blessed, live joyfully, and accept my congratulations on your remarkable journey.

# EMOTIONAL ANATOMY

Effective therapists acknowledge the role of emotions in healing. Our job in the future may be to more fully investigate the slowdown of energy our clients present us, the *why* of that slowdown, and the *how* of taking the client back into and through the slowdown by whatever means is appropriate and effective to create physical health. Skillful and careful listening begins this process naturally. In other words, effective work may be more about the intention to elicit and facilitate release and less about training, replication or duplication of results, or quick fixes. It's simple, but it's not easy.

Certain diseases, symptoms, postures, and patterns may correspond to specific emotions or reactions to situations. The following ideas are just that: ideas and guidelines, not a written-in-stone textbook! Yet a person with a depressed stance may eventually become depressed. A girl who develops breasts or height before her classmates will probably try to shrink in height and hide her chest, possibly leading to breast cancer, a heart condition, shoulder and arm problems, or headaches.

Let's again consider wisdom from classical Oriental medicine. Qi or chi boils when one is angry (chakra 5), but weakens when one is fearful (chakra 1), sad (chakra 4), or mentally disturbed or fatigued (chakra 6). Any stagnation or imbalance of chi causes health challenges—the slowdown of energy.

Recognition of emotional symptoms can help a client release them. By pointing out the neck could let go—and perhaps asking, "So, who's your pain in the neck?"—you've given the client a gift. Possibly they weren't yet aware of their degree of holding. Our job becomes to identify or help the client identify the holding; and through manipulation, verbal and non-verbal, stretching, and breathwork, to let go of these holdings. Many people will tell you they're "fine": Feelings Internalized, Not Expressed.

Louise Hay's book *You Can Heal Your Life* (1984) is an excellent reference point with which to start investigating emotional anatomy. Her ideas seem a good jumping-off point. In her model, the root of most sickness is the belief "I'm not good enough," which manifests in some fear-based emotion: fear, shame, indecision, anger, grief, mental confusion, or unhappiness. All these negative emotions work the same way: they shorten the body in fear instead of lengthening and allowing energy to flow through us. While I don't tend to believe any condition is always caused by a specific stimulus, these ideas are worth considering. Though I've been advised by some to delete this appendix, I still feel it has worthwhile information and new ideas for some to consider.

I also like Dr. Christiane Northrup's (2010) view that any illness condition is merely a form of meditation—in other words, if we don't take time to find quiet and meditate, our bodies will find a way for us to get our time out. So here are some of my ideas as to why we create, or accept, conditions in our bodies:

## EMOTIONAL ANATOMY GLOSSARY

**Accidents** Why are you self-sabotaging? There are no accidents. Why are you not in the moment, but in the future or past? This is a misstatement of your place in space and time.

**Acne** Self-dislike. Lack of acceptance of self, others, or current situations.

**Adrenals** Extremely run down, defeated, or anxious. Out of juice from pouring on the power for too long without rest.

**Alzheimer's** The mental files are full and he or she refuses to clean them. The early mental files are manageable, but the new ones are overwhelming.

**Aneurism** Brain: mental overworking. Aortic: physical underworking.

**Ankles** Represent flexibility and moving forward in life. They should be hinged, joyous, and vigorous. We plod.

**Arches** Flat feet: being overcared for, often by mother—too much safety and no challenge in the world. High arches: not enough safety—essence sucked in all the way to the stomach.

**Arms** Represent reaching out for our good, receiving it, holding it, and sharing it.

**Arthritis** Critical self- or other-directed thoughts. Can't let the joy flow through.

**Asthma** Smother love. Stifled, often by an overprotective mother. Belief that the world is unsafe.

**Back** Erectors hold us up even when we really don't feel like standing up for ourselves. The pain comes from having to brace ourselves against the world instead of letting life flow through. Upper and middle are often about guilt and fear; low can be money worries and sexual fears. Digging in your heels is the number one cause of back problems. Also, remember that, whether you feel back pain in the upper, lower, or middle, chances are the entire spine is involved in the pattern.

**Blood pressure** High: allowing stresses of life to run your life, and struggling. Low: allowing stresses of life to defeat you. Surrender.

**Brain** Mental governor; too much going on mentally.

**Breast** Nourishment and protection. Not allowing self to nurture or be nurtured. Closing down the heart so as to not feel the pain.

**Bronchitis** Belief it's not safe to take a deep breath. Inflamed family environment.

**Bursitis** Inflammation due to overuse with underappreciation.

**Buttocks** Tight buttocks say "I'm in control (but I fear I may lose it)."

**Cancer** Deep grief over a real or perceived loss, usually occurring one to two years after the loss. Cancer patients are often good sufferers and model patients who believe they've gotten over their grief.

**Carpal** Performance anxiety. Forgetting to relax and breathe in the need to achieve. Overuse and overachieving.

**Colds** Being worn down by too many stressors, then when the light at the end is visible, relaxing into collapse. The immune system relaxes and gets overpowered.

**Colon** Moves nutrition through, or holds on from fear of lack.

**Constipation** Can't let go of old ways. Paralysis regarding looking ahead. Can't process and eliminate ideas.

**Depression** What's the use? I can never measure up/be enough. Anger/hopelessness turned inward.

**Diabetes** Don't believe one can or should enjoy the sweetness of life.

**Eyes/ears** What is it you don't want to see or hear?

**Fat** Protection. "I'll just hide down here at the center of me, and be safe and invisible." Or, "I'll dilute the churning in my guts by putting more into them."

**Feet** Our foundation, understanding, and direction in life. How solid are we?

**Fibromyalgia** Life has taken the wind out of my sails, and I can't get my breath back…good sufferers and achievers.

**Hands/fingers** Reaching out and touching, creating. Hands are the outmost extension of the heart line.

**Headaches** Fear of losing control, so shortening the head and neck. Pulling into your turtle shell. Or, someone or something, negative or unresolved, has attached to you at the back of the head.

**Heart** Master organ, center of safety and joy. Problems are about inability to find and express joy, love, purpose, and flow in one's life.

**Heels** Defenders of the core line; we dig in our heels to stand our ground.

**Hips** Moving forward into life. Fear of procreation or sexual enjoyment.

**Jaw** Biting off harsh words and self-censoring. Biting the tongue and holding anger in, instead of telling someone off.

**Kidney** Pissed off…holding onto too much of mental and physical toxicity. In Oriental medicine Kidney qi is nearly always deficient in today's world, as is the adrenal system directly above it. Many of us place a protective shell over our backs in this kidney area.

**Knees** Direction. Indecision about where forward actually is. Not knowing where you truly want to go, or sometimes stubbornness (locked knees).

**Left side** Represents feminine or mother energy.

**Legs** Move us forward into the future. Shutting down legs is like a tree dying from the roots, not letting earth energy up and through.

**Liver** Anger. Stored toxicities of the physical or emotional variety. Unprocessed feelings that fester.

**Lungs** Accepting life, breathing in and living in joy. Need to grieve satisfyingly.

**Menstrual** Inability to allow the feminine to flow through. Self-punishment or belief that menstruation is unclean and must be painful and endured since it can't be stopped.

**Neck** Inflexibility, stubbornness, fear of change. Pulling your head into a shell.

**Pain** A signal something's out of balance. Ida Rolf said, "Pain is resistance to change." I'd add that pain is resistance to change that comes too quickly.

**Pancreas** Need for sweetness in one's life.

**Prostate** Not accepting or being comfortable with the male role, or being made to feel powerless.

**Psoriasis** Core takes all the energy, so none left for the sleeve.

**Right side** Represents masculine or father energy.

**Sciatica** Holding on for dear life, digging in your heels: fear of money issues, not being good enough, or needing to stand your ground.

**Scoliosis** Not being allowed to express the way you want, to stand up for self. Being under someone's thumb (often the mother).

**Sex dysfunction** Self-punishment or turning off the sexual feelings due to abuse, poorly received attempts to be sexual, or trained to believe sexual feelings are shameful.

**Shoulders** Life is a burden: How do we carry it? By shrinking we can get smaller, and make a smaller target. Holding shoulders rigidly can indicate stuck qi or chi. They're ready for a fight.

**Spine** Shrinking and shortening in response to fear. Trying to stand up and meet others' expectations.

**Spleen** Needing to "vent" anger and allow emotions to achieve balance.

**Stomach** Fear, undigested thoughts and feelings. Difficulty in processing, accepting, and eliminating that in our life which comes at us and through us.

**Thighs** Weariness. "These have carried me long enough."

**Throat** Creativity and expression issues. "Swallowing" anger or pride. May also be an indicator of sexual abuse.

**Thyroid** Rationing out of joy—we can't have too much, because that would be unsafe.

**Toes** The spring that powers forward progress or gives up in de-feet.

**Tongue** Connects to the deepest line of the body and censors self instead of expressing. Sometimes grief stored under the tongue.

**Tumors** Energetic slowdowns or cysts: unfulfilled desires.

**Ulcers** What's eating you up? Anger, fear, shame turned inward and eating at you.

**Varicosities** Feeling static and losing the spring in step and joy in life.

# THE FACES OF FEAR

At the suggestion of my students I created a working paper which goes in the other direction: Which emotions lead to specific conditions? While this is the beginning of a work that some of you may find valueless, I think it's interesting to see that various faces of fear may take slightly different directions in our bodymind's quest to shut down, not look, and suffer rather than do the cleaning work we need. Keep in mind, these are ideas. You can add your own, or see other correlations entirely.

One last note: None of these fear-based emotions is by itself a bad thing. Being stuck in a fear-based emotion is an unhealthy condition. Personally I believe so is being stuck in any emotion including joy, love, and satisfaction. In my world, experience the emotion and let it go.

**Abandonment/alone/afraid** Can lead to Alzheimer's. It's a necessity of a healthy human to have someone to process/debrief/de-stress with. When we lose this person, or never find them, we sink farther into ourselves, shrinking out the universe. This can also lead to depression, cancer, and arthritis.

**Anger** Anger turned inward can cause depression. Anger not expressed can inflame the heart and contribute to digestive problems, ulcers, and bipolar disorder. Anger disturbs the Liver qi. One may see symptoms in the head and neck: headaches, blotches, or a red face.

**Fear** The paralysis of fear can lead us to forgetting to breathe and flow. This can cause fibromyalgia and chronic fatigue syndrome. Digestive disorders also seem to come from undigested fear, which also affects the Kidney meridian. Anxiety, sleeplessness, and a pounding heart may be symptoms of fear.

**Frustrated, misunderstood, hurt** These emotions cause one to feel unheard or invalidated. They can lead to TMJ, throat issues, bronchitis, and digestive (again!) problems.

**Grief** Unprocessed grief needs to be acknowledged, otherwise it may manifest as cancer, throat issues, and lung problems.

**Guilt** Guilt weighs more heavily than perhaps any emotion, causing us to spin our wheels mentally. Like alone/afraid, when we feel guilty we hold ourselves in; unprocessed thoughts can lead to mental disorders.

**Resentment** Holding onto feelings of jealousy or competition can manifest arthritis or pain throughout the body.

**Sadness** Can bring us depression, CFS, fibromyalgia, cancer, etc. Sadness is a deadly slowdown of energy that causes us to shut down life tremendously. It depletes qi, weakens the lungs, and affects the heart. Conversely, excessive joy makes the heart act erratically.

**Shame** Shame tends to make us want to shorten down and take up less space. Posturally we can go into kyphosis (stooping) which contributes to heart congestion, fibro, and panic or anxiety disorders.

**Shock** An outer shock shrinks the core, draws the qi inward and disrupts Heart and Small Intestine meridians, and depletes the heart.

**Unworthiness** To Louise Hay (and to me) this is the root of most disease. I particularly think unworthiness contributes to heart problems, stomach problems, and diabetes (sweetness of life) issues.

**Worry** *Worthless, Old, Rotten, Recycled Yap.* Excess thinking is like spinning one's wheels and exhausts the spleen. This person might be served by slowing down and paying attention to mealtimes as relaxation and recharging instead of a time to do more business.

# BIBLIOGRAPHY AND SUGGESTED READINGS

The following books may provide additional ideas and information to you that support your quest to become a more effective therapist. I've given information about publishers, etc., but also a distillation of the ideas each book presents that may make you want to investigate it.

## ANATOMY TEXTS

Biel, Andrew: *Trail Guide to the Body* (Books of Discovery, Boulder, CO, 1997).

A fairly new and comprehensive look at the body...currently one of the best for therapists.

Cross, John R.: *Acupuncture and the Chakra Energy System: Treating the Cause of Disease* (North Atlantic Books, Berkeley, CA, 2008).

I like the concept of contrasting the chakra system with the meridian system.

Egoscue, Pete: *Pain Free: A Revolutionary Method for Stopping Chronic Pain* (Bantam Books, New York, 1998).

This is a wonderful book to get you thinking about looking at the entire deep line of the body and how to align it posturally to make function cleaner and happier.

Endo, Ryokyu: *Tao Shiatsu: Life Medicine for the 21st Century* (Japan Publications, Tokyo and New York, 1995).

A really great guide to how Eastern medicine works to restore the energy of the individual and the energy exchange between the individual and nature.

Feitis, Rosemary: *Ida Rolf Talks About Rolfing and Physical Reality* (Healing Arts Press, Rochester, VT, 1990).

This is Ida Rolf's philosophy. Many of us could enjoy reading the whys and wherefores that let us know how she came to her conclusions.

Findlay, Susan: *Sports Massage* (Human Kinetics, Champaign, IL, 2010).

A concise and basic guide of techniques to give good deep tissue work, full of illustrations.

Heller, Joseph and Henkin, William A.: *Bodywise: An Introduction to Hellerwork for Regaining Flexibility and Wellbeing* (North Atlantic Books, Berkeley, CA, 2004).

If one wanted to get the Ida Rolf recipe for ten sessions, Heller nearly gives it away in this book, along with his own twists on deep work.

Kapit, Wynn and Elson, Lawrence M.: *Anatomy Coloring Book* (HarperCollins, New York, 1993).

A standard and wonderful way to renew your anatomy skills by returning to the basic drawings of anatomy and physiology.

Myers, Tom: *Anatomy Trains* (Churchill Livingstone, Edinburgh and London, 2001).

Tom has done great work in creating fascial roadmaps to tie seemingly unconnected problems in the body together, to assist us in letting them release from each other.

Netter, Frank: *Atlas of Human Anatomy* (Saunders/Elsevier, Philadelphia, PA, 1989).

The best pictures of tissue I've seen.

Northrup, Christiane: *Women's Bodies, Women's Wisdom: Creating Physical and Emotional Health and Healing* (Bantam Books, New York, 2010).

While written primarily as a guide to health for women, this book is full of commonsense ideas that could enhance anyone's health.

Pallardy, Pierre: *Gut Instinct: What Your Stomach Is Trying to Tell You* (Rodale International, London, 2006).

An interesting theory that everything in the body can be healed by attention to the gut.

Riggs, Art: *Deep Tissue Massage* (North Atlantic Books, Berkeley, CA, 2002).

A very good guide to the specific deep tissue technique.

Rolf, Ida: *Rolfing: The Integration of Human Structure* (Harper & Row, New York, Hagerstown, San Francisco, and London, 1977).

This is Ida Rolf's textbook. While it won't teach you to become a Rolfer in ten easy lessons, it will give you a good insight into a great mind.

Schultz, Louis: *The Endless Web: Fascial Anatomy and Physical Reality* (Schultz, Feitis, Salles, and Thompson; North Atlantic Books, Berkeley, CA, 1996).

My mentor Louis has written what I think is simply the best book about fascia and what it does.

Warfel, John H.: *The Extremities* and *The Head, Neck and Trunk* (Lea & Fabiger, Philadelphia, PA, 1974).

I like the simplicity of these two little books: each muscle has its own page of a simple line drawing with the origin/insertion/innervations/blood supply/function given for each.

## SELF-HELP BOOKS

Bond, Mary: *Rolfing Movement Integration* (Healing Arts Press, Rochester, VT, 1993).

My clients have always enjoyed working with Bond's ideas for learning to live in and move their bodies more appropriately.

Bond, Mary: *The New Rules of Posture* (Healing Arts Press, Rochester, VT, 2007).

This more recent Bond book continues to encourage clients to learn to honor, listen to, stretch, and use their bodies more efficiently.

Gentry, Byron with Gentry, Mary: *Miracles of the Mind: How to Use the Power of Your Mind for Healing and Prosperity* (Rainbow Books, Highland City, FL, 1998).

Another of my mentors, Gentry created a specific formula designed to harness mental, physical, and emotional energy to create health in clients.

Hay, Louise: *You Can Heal Your Life (You Can Heal Your Body)* (Hay House, Santa Monica, CA, 1984).

Hay believes the root of disease is lack of self-esteem, and gives a good glossary of conditions and illnesses with both causes and affirmations to help unwind them.

Karrasch, Noah: *Meet Your Body: CORE Bodywork and Rolfing Tools to Release Bodymindcore Trauma* (Singing Dragon, London and Philadelphia, 2009).

This book is primarily for clients, giving them many ideas for maintaining ease in their own bodies.

Myss, Caroline and Shealy, C. Norman, MD: *The Creation of Health: The Emotional, Psychological, and Spiritual Responses That Promote Health and Healing* (Three Rivers Press, New York, 1998).

Caroline and Norm look at many case studies and readings of patients and draw interesting conclusions. Look for "Jonah's" story in this book.

Painter, Jack: *Deep Bodywork and Personal Development: Harmonizing Our Bodies, Emotions and Thoughts* (Bodymind, Olympia, WA, 1986).

Painter has thought deeply about the connection between emotions and illness or pain. This book is a good primer for those interested in changing thinking.

Pierrakos, Eva: *The Pathwork of Self Transformation* (Bantam New Age, New York, 1990).

The message of this book seems to me to be simply, "Feel your feelings."

Pierrakos, John: *CORE Energetics: Developing the Capacity to Love and Heal* (Core Evolution, Mendocino, CA, 2005).

A gem. Pierrakos challenges us all to allow our core or essence to interact through our body with our environment.

Ponder, Catherine: *Open Your Mind to Prosperity* (DeVorss & Co, Marina Del Ray, CA, 1984).

Another book on prosperity is never a bad idea; I like Ponder's statement that congestion is the culprit, always.

Truman, Karol Kuhn: *Feelings Buried Alive Never Die* (self published, UT, 1991).

Now a standard text for those interested in learning to deal with feelings instead of pretending they're bad or don't exist.

## PHILOSOPHY

Becker, Robert O. and Selden, Gary: *The Body Electric: Electromagnetism and the Foundation of Life* (William Morrow, New York, 1998).

Beginning with the question "How do salamanders regenerate missing pieces?" Becker traces the development of the realization of energy fields.

Brennan, Barbara: *Hands of Light* (Bantam Books, New York, 1988).

Brennan attempts to communicate energy medicine to the medical community with this book. Some wonderful illustrations of auras and energy bodies.

Dossey, Larry: *Healing Words: The Power of Prayer and the Practice of Medicine* (Harper One, New York, 1995).

Setting out to prove that prayer wasn't effective in healing, scientist Dossey was surprised.

Emoto, Masuru: *Heal Thyself: The Message from Water III* (Hay House, Carlsbad, CA, 2004).

This amazing book shows photos of magnified water: the more positive energy surrounding the water, the more crystalline the structure, and the more negative energy surrounding the water, the more chaotic the structure. And we are what percent water in our bodies?

Frank, Jerome and Frank, Julia: *Persuasion and Healing* (Johns Hopkins University Press, Boston, MA, 1961).

A rather scholarly work that deals with the cause and treatment of mental illness from a psychiatrist's viewpoint. Some real nuggets in a rather chewy book.

Frankl, Viktor: *Man's Search for Meaning* (Beacon Press, Boston, MA, 1959).

After observing prisoners of war in Nazi concentration camps, Frankl realized that those who found purpose in their lives, positive or negative, lived longer. It allows us to see how health relates to living "on purpose."

Forni, P.M.: *Choosing Civility: The Twenty-Five Rules of Considerate Conduct* (St. Martin's Griffin, New York, 2002).

Forni's simplest definition of civility is "benevolent awareness of others." Lots to think about for all of us, especially therapists.

Hillman, James: *The Soul's Code: In Search of Character and Calling* (Bantam Books, London, 1997).

Suggests that each soul has a specific path to fulfill: health comes when we are happily on that path.

Lipton, Bruce: *The Biology of Belief* (Mountain of Love, Marina del Rey, CA, 2008).

Lipton says that although DNA can't be totally altered, we also have an on/off switch that allows us to alter behaviors, and therefore physiology.

Myss, Caroline: *Anatomy of the Spirit* (Three Rivers Press, New York, 1996).

In this book Myss manages to overlay the chakra system on Christian sacraments and Jewish tenets. Thought-provoking.

Oschmann, Jim: *Energy Medicine: The Scientific Basis* (Elsevier, Philadelphia, PA, 2000).

A good historical perspective of the understanding and practice of energy medicine through the ages.

Pert, Candace: *Molecules of Emotion* (Touchstone, New York, 1997).

Pert was the first scientist to say our emotions affect our physiology at the cellular level.

Snowdon, David: *Aging with Grace: What the Nun Story Teaches Us about Leading Longer, Healthier, More Meaningful Lives* (Bantam Books, New York, 2001).

A fascinating study showing us that, while Alzheimer's disease may live in the tissues, it may not necessarily affect the mind when a person is determined to stay current with the larger world.

Tompkins, Peter and Bird, Christopher: *The Secret Life of Plants* (Harper & Row, New York, 1973).

A summary of interesting research with plants, showing they do have consciousness.

Wu, Master Zhongxian: *Seeking the Spirit of the Book of Change* (Singing Dragon, London and Philadelphia, 2009).

This nearly indescribable book invites one to explore Chinese traditions around medicine, divination, and life.

# INDEX